Physical Exercise Interventions for Mental Health

Contents

Contributors

David A. Baron MSEd DO, Department of Psychiatry, Keck Hospital at USC; Director, Global Center for Exercise, Psychiatry and Sport at USC; Keck School of Medicine, University of Southern California, Los Angeles, CA, USA

Steven H. Baron PhD, Montgomery County Community College, Blue Bell, PA, USA

Eric Chen MD, Department of Psychiatry, Queen Mary Hospital, University of Hong Kong, Hong Kong, China

Kay L. Cox MD, School of Medicine and Pharmacology, University of Western Australia, Crawley, WA, Australia

Richard R. Dopp MD, Department of Psychiatry, University of Michigan, Ann Arbor, MI, USA

Shantel L. Duffy MD, Healthy Brain Ageing Program, Brain and Mind Research Institute, University of Sydney, Sydney, NSW, Australia

Peter Falkai MD, Department of Psychiatry and Psychotherapy, Ludwig Maximilian University, Munich, Bavaria, Germany

Barry A. Franklin PhD, Cardiac Rehabilitation and Exercise Laboratories, Division of Cardiology, William Beaumont Hospital, Royal Oak, MI, USA

B. N. Gangadhar MD DSc, NIMHANS Integrated Centre for Yoga, Department of Psychiatry, National Institute of Mental Health and Neurosciences, Bengaluru, Karnataka, India

Tracy L. Greer PhD, Department of Psychiatry, UT Southwestern Medical Center, Dallas, TX, USA

Linda C. W. Lam MD, Department of Psychiatry, Chinese University of Hong Kong, Hong Kong, China

Amit Lampit MD, Regenerative Neuroscience Group, Brain and Mind Research Institute, University of Sydney, Sydney, NSW, Australia

Samantha Lasarow BA, Stanford University, Stanford, CA, USA

Nicola T. Lautenschlager MD, Academic Unit for Psychiatry of Old Age, Department of Psychiatry, The University of Melbourne & NorthWestern Mental Health, Melbourne Health, Melbourne, Australia

Edwin Lee FHKCPsych, Department of Psychiatry, Queen Mary Hospital, University of Hong Kong, Hong Kong, China

Sing Lee FHKCPsych, Department of Psychiatry, Chinese University of Hong Kong, Hong Kong, China

Jessie Lin, Department of Psychiatry, Queen Mary Hospital, University of Hong Kong, Hong Kong, China

Arthur D. P. Mak FHKCPsych, Department of Psychiatry, Chinese University of Hong Kong, Hong Kong, China

Berend Malchow MD, Department of Psychiatry and Psychotherapy, Ludwig Maximilian University, Munich, Bavaria, Germany

Chad D. Rethorst PhD, Department of Psychiatry, UT Southwestern Medical Center, Dallas, TX, USA

Andrea Schmitt MD, Department of Psychiatry and Psychotherapy, Ludwig Maximilian University, Munich, Bavaria, Germany

Bradley L. Stilger MD, Department of Psychiatry, University of Michigan, Ann Arbor, MI, USA

Justin E. Trivax MD, Division of Cardiology, William Beaumont Hospital, Royal Oak, MI, USA

Madhukar H. Trivedi MD, Betty Jo Hay Distinguished Chair in Mental Health, and Comprehensive Center for Depression, UT Southwestern Medical Center, Dallas, TX, USA

Michael Valenzuela MD, Regenerative Neuroscience Group, Brain and Mind Research Institute, University of Sydney, Sydney, NSW, Australia

Thomas E. Vanhecke MD, Division of Cardiology, William Beaumont Hospital, Royal Oak, MI, USA

Shivarama Varambally MD, NIMHANS Integrated Centre for Yoga, Department of Psychiatry, National Institute of Mental Health and Neurosciences, Bengaluru, Karnataka, India

Foreword

The authors and editors of Physical Exercise Interventions for Mental Health have presented a comprehensive framework of recent research on physical exercise interventions for different mental health conditions. The book is prepared with integration on current research evidence, and supplemented with invaluable experience by academic clinicians in this area.

It is acknowledged that management of mental health problems is highly complex. The need for a perceptive approach towards different treatment paradigms with careful scrutiny through current scientific methods should not be under-emphasized. This book helps to inform readers about available evidence through reviews of clinical trials and experiments on basic science. Physical exercise interventions appeared to provide support for its therapeutic efficacy in various dimensions of impairments for different mental conditions across the life span. Authors in the book outlined its potential mechanisms underlying apparent improvement for different conditions, which converge to the integrity of brain function through pathways affecting neurochemical and neurophysiological balances. Their translation of this 'well known' life activity into a 'scientific and clinical concept' with clear guidelines will help many health care professionals who wish to include physical exercise into their practice protocols.

Linda C. W. Lam, MD
Michelle Riba, MD

Recent developments of physical activity interventions as an adjuvant therapy in mental disorders

Linda C. W. Lam

Mental disorders are prevalent and disabling conditions. Major epidemiologic studies reveal that from 10% to over 30% of the adult population suffers from mood disorders with depression and anxiety (Kessler et al., 2005). More severe mental disorders, typically represented as schizophrenia and related psychoses, are represented in about 1% of the population worldwide. The Global Burden of Disease Study 2010 (GBD, 2010) estimated that a substantial proportion of the world's disease burden comes from mental, neurological and substance-use disorders. Mental disorders cause the most significant disability-adjusted life years (DALYs) for chronic conditions in adulthood (Whiteford et al., 2015). In the adult population, mental disorders not only cause loss of productivity and disability, they also increase the risks of early mortality as a result of self-harm behaviours and co-morbid physical disorders.

Etiological factors of mental disorders are extremely complex. Constitutional predispositions, genetic factors, early life experiences, personality, psychosocial stressors and physical health all contribute to symptom development and affect disease course across the life span. In contrast, our understanding of the patho-logical mechanisms related to mental disorders is still very limited. Recognized treatments for different mental disorders have relied on empirical evidence of a few pharmacological and psychological interventions. Comprehensive theoretical support for the standard intervention has not yet been able to fully explain the physiological impact of available interventions.

Psychotropic medication brings satisfactory improvement to disturbing symptoms of most mental disorders. Psychosocial interventions, especially specific types of psychotherapy, including cognitive behavioural therapy and mindfulness-based cognitive therapy, have been found to offer significant benefits to those suffering from depression. However, satisfactory outcomes from clinical trials frequently do not translate to full recovery. Residual symptoms are not

Physical Exercise Interventions for Mental Health, ed. Linda C. W. Lam and Michelle Riba. Published by Cambridge University Press. © Cambridge University Press 2016.

uncommon, and many people experience relapses of symptoms after the initial remission. There is a definite need to explore additional approaches that may augment the therapeutic efficacy of conventional treatments. It would be even better if new approaches could enrich and expand the available intervention paradigms.

Mental disorders reflect disturbances in brain function

It is well recognized that the aberrant psychological experiences in mental disorders are closely linked to disturbances in brain function. Hypotheses have been developed around the major neurotransmitter pathways, which are implicated in different psychiatric symptoms. These hypotheses have formed the basis of pharmacological interventions. Serotonin and noradrenaline are postulated to be associated with depression and anxiety, while dopamine and N-methyl-D-aspartate (NMDA) are associated with psychotic-like symptoms. Genetic studies have revealed that most mental disorders, psychoses and bipolar affective disorders in particular are associated with constitutional predispositions that impose constitutional risk states. Many of the gene loci associated with mental disorders are related to neurotransmitter and immune pathways (Schizophrenia Working Group of the Psychiatric Genomics Consortium, 2014).

Neuroimaging studies further suggest that structural abnormality of the brain is found in persons with mental disorders. Cerebral atrophy and ventricular dilatation have been well recognized in different forms of dementia. In the past few decades, it has also been demonstrated that schizophrenia is associated with atrophy of temporal and frontal lobes as early as a few years after disease onset. Advances in functional neuroimaging have brought further insights into the abnormal brain connectivity associated with mental disorders.

In the past hundred years, our concepts about mental disorders have evolved from a mystic background to psychosocial theories. With further appreciation of the neurological underpinnings of functional brain abnormalities, clinicians have become increasingly interested in developing treatment approaches that will attenuate brain disturbance and hopefully restore functional impairments.

Physical exercise as a possible treatment option

It is common knowledge that exercise is important for the maintenance of good physical health. Nor is the appreciation of physical exercise as beneficial for mental wellbeing and disease conditions a new idea. However, unlike guidelines for cardiovascular fitness, physical exercise as a treatment for mental disorders has never been formally studied on an experimental basis so that it may be incorporated into routine clinical advice and practice. We still lack sufficient empirical evidence. Nor have we developed comprehensive conceptual frameworks relating the neural mechanism of physical exercise. These problems hinder the integration of specific physical exercise programs as standard therapy. Additionally, the motivational and emotional disturbances associated with mental disorders hinder patients from adhering to exercise programs.

There has been an upsurge of interest in research on physical exercise and mental health. This has been greatly aided by advancements in the understanding of neurophysiological mechanisms underlying physical activity. Evidence that regular physical activities effect brain changes can now be considered from the perspective of alterations in physiological response, such as the increase in brain-derived neurotrophic factor (BDNF) during physical exercise. There is converging opinion that exercise interventions bring about brain changes in structures and connectivity. Advances in neuroscience techniques are bringing new dimensions to the subject, adding scientific rigour and substance to further propose that physical exercise be comprehensively evaluated as a treatment strategy for mental disorders. For health practitioners, there are frequently many questions to be answered before advising patients with different mental conditions on the proper exercise regime for their conditions. Given such highly individualized needs, it may be over-simplistic to set up a one-size-fits-all recommendation. In contrast, it is important to adopt a conceptual framework which guides practice.

This book helps mental-health professionals and clinicians revisit the current research on physical exercise and its effectiveness for the treatment of mental disorders. Apart from reviewing the updated findings of clinical trials, the authors also highlight how the mechanisms of physical exercise modulate neuroplastic responses. Most importantly, practical advice is given about implementing exercise regimes for clients with mood, psychosis and cognitive disorders. The authors discuss the choice of exercise, start-up schedules and motivational and personal factors. The central theme is to develop tailor-made approaches.

Physical exercise interventions for mood disorders

Depression and anxiety disorders are extremely common in every community. These conditions are disturbing because the symptoms cause significant psychological distress and impair productivity and interpersonal relationships. These complex disease-modulating factors call for a multi-dimensional approach to management. For many decades, medication and psychological interventions have been gaining popularity and have been recognized as mainstay treatments for mental disorders. However, there is definitely room for further improvement.

Research in health psychology suggests that physical exercise may produce acute anxiolytic effects after exercise. However, very few large-scale randomized controlled clinical trials have been specially conducted to examine the effects of physical exercise on different anxiety disorders. Chapter 6, on physical exercise and anxiety, examines the current evidence of beneficial effects of physical exercise in individuals with constitutional anxiety sensitivity and specific anxiety disorders. The impact of exercise on calming nerves appears to be best conceptualized through a broad and diverse approach that includes behavioural adaptation, autonomic nervous regulation, social support and neurophysiological alterations. To treat the core symptoms of anxiety specifically, diverse modalities of exercise interventions including mind-body approaches and breathing exercises are alternative options to conventional aerobic approaches in physical health.

Major depressive disorder (MDD) is another highly prevalent condition that ranks near the top in disease burden. The development of antidepressants has brought about satisfactory responses in many people. However, recurrences and incomplete remission are not uncommon. Aerobic exercise has been recognised for its mood-elevating effects with supporting evidence by associated neurophysiological changes. In Chapter 3, which addresses physical exercise and depression, Baron and his colleagues have provided a succinct review of the evidence of physical exercise interventions in the treatment of depression, with case studies to illustrate how exercise can have therapeutic effects on mood in different clinical contexts. In Chapter 11, Stilger and colleagues explain the significance of adjuvant exercise intervention to optimize depressive symptoms, as they elaborate on the associations between exercise, depression and cardiovascular diseases. Concurrent depression significantly affects the prognosis of cardiovascular conditions. It worsens disease severity, hinders rehabilitation and is associated with significantly higher mortality. Although complex interactive mechanisms are important in explaining how disease courses cross-over, physical exercise provides a useful therapeutic bridge for both depression and cardiovascular disease, making it an attractive option for treatment.

It is unclear as to the dosage and intensity of aerobic exercise for good antidepressant effect. In Chapter 7, Rethorst and his colleagues have detailed the implementation of the Treatment with Exercise Augmentation for Depression (TREAD) study, highlighting the comparison between high and low doses of aerobic exercise in alleviating depressed mood and various associated symptoms. Comprehensive and in-depth analyses of different clinical outcomes hint that individual characteristics, including family history of depression and physical health status, are important modulators for treatment response. This highlights the need for good understanding of biological mechanisms so that tailor-made approaches can be developed.

MDD in adolescents is an even more complicated condition. Conventional antidepressants are associated with adverse effects, which makes them less popular treatments. Psychosocial interventions, by contrast, are less well established in this age group. Physical exercise intervention is an attractive option. It has a high safety profile and is more user-friendly to young people. In Chapter 2, Dopp outlines the study of physical exercise interventions and the encouraging preliminary evidence that they may be useful add-ons or independent therapies for adolescents with MDD.

New directions to augment management regimes for schizophrenia and related psychosis

Schizophrenia is one of the most disabling illnesses in adult life. Positive symptoms of hallucinations and delusions are not only dreadful life experiences, but also lead to impaired judgement and risks. Fortunately, these symptoms are effectively managed by pharmacological interventions. Affective dysregulation, cognitive impairment and loss of volition are more prominent in the chronic stage of the disease. They are associated with a deficit state that limits recovery and integration into the community. Unfortunately, these symptoms have not been managed effectively with available treatment options, such as medication and psychotherapy. Over the years, various attempts have been developed with specific strategies for management of the cognitive and motivational deficits of schizophrenia, but success is still far from near. Popular use of second-generation antipsychotic medication in the past decades has alerted clinicians of the need to treat the metabolic side effects and increased body weight, which are unwanted side effects of these drugs. This necessitates attention to the need to implement adjuvant physical exercise intervention in people taking medication for the treatment of psychosis. There is ample evidence to suggest that early introduction of aerobic exercise regime is efficacious in reducing metabolic side effects.

The story becomes richer through our current understanding of the neurophysiological basis of schizophrenic psychosis in the neurotransmitter, immune and inflammatory pathway. Physical exercise, especially aerobic exercise, appears to have potential in optimizing neuroprotective reactions, and hopefully it could recalibrate the dampened neuroplastic responses. In Chapter 5, Malchow and his colleagues have detailed recent advances in exercise interventions in schizophrenic psychosis, focusing on the positive structural and functional brain changes that take place with intervention. Considerations on different modalities of exercise are also laid out to assist readers for consideration in treatment planning.

Because schizophrenic psychosis is a chronic and relapsing illness and cognitive deficits start early, it is imperative to evaluate whether exercise interventions should start at the earliest phase of illness. In Chapter 4, on physical exercise for early psychosis, Chen and Lee have shared their own experiences with exercise intervention in young adults with first-episode psychosis, and they discuss the challenges involved in researching and promoting exercise intervention for this group. The authors also introduce the Hong Kong–based FitMind program for people recovering from psychotic episodes. They elaborate on the barriers and facilitators for successful implementation of exercise-based interventions for persons in the community recovering from first-onset psychotic episode.

Activity for the developing and ageing brain – impact of exercise on cognition

Researchers who are attracted to studies on physical exercise for mental disorders are keen to further their understanding of the neural basis underlying physical exercise. This is especially relevant when one considers the different mental disorders that span the life course. For neurodevelopmental disorders with onset in childhood, such as autistic spectrum disorder and attention deficit hyperactivity disorder, specific cognitive deficits are the core features leading to functional disabilities and difficulty in learning. With increasing awareness of the problem, there is a definite need to develop non-invasive and safe strategies to augment brain function in this special population with maturing brains. In Chapter 2, Dopp introduces studies of exercise interventions for different neurodevelopmental disorders and discusses the preliminary evidence of feasibility and possible symptom improvements in these conditions.

At the other end of the life cycle, population ageing is a worldwide trend. The inevitable consequence of longevity is the increasing prevalence of dementia and other neurocognitive disorders. The World Health Organization considers dementia a public health priority. Although we may have gained much understanding of the pathological mechanisms and disease-modulating factors in the major types of dementia in late life, there have been great delays and disappointments in drug development. In the past decade, potentially promising clinical trials, built on pathological models of Alzheimer's disease, have mostly failed to reach satisfactory clinical outcomes. Available treatment options are only of very limited therapeutic efficacy. No approved drug can effectively slow down the trajectory of cognitive or functional decline in persons suffering from dementia. Repeated epidemiological and cohort studies, however, have found that lifestyles offer protective effects in cognition. Assumption of regular physical activities is found to be associated with lower risks of developing dementia. It is hypothesized that exercise will enhance the neuroplastic response, offering some protective responses against continuous degeneration. In Chapter 10, Lampit and his colleagues examine the translational perspective of physical exercise on cognition. The authors have examined the model linking physical exercise and cognition, and have specifically evaluated evidence of frontal-executive and hippocampal response to exercise intervention. In the review of animal studies, they discuss the significance of environmental stimulation and enrichment in optimizing cognition through exercise. As with all forms of psychosocial intervention, therapeutic factors are frequently inter-related and need to be considered within a holistic perspective.

Lifestyle changes are hard to introduce and even more difficult to consolidate and sustain. The barriers are particularly high for older adults with compromised cognition and mental functioning, in addition to their concomitant physical frailty. In Chapter 8, Lautenschlager and Cox draw on their rich experience of clinical trials in mild cognitive impairment and dementia, and offer step-by-step guidance on starting exercise intervention. They carefully evaluate advice about the modality of exercise and logistics of intervention and the psychological factors that enhance motivation for long-term adherence. Self-efficacy, social support, skills learning, self-regulation and goal setting are indispensable components for ensuring successful integration into personal habits, which can only offer benefits in the long run. This practitioner's guide will certainly be welcomed by frontline professionals whose patients are requesting specific instructions as to what to do and how to start.

Does only aerobic exercise work?

The recommendation of the American Heart Association of 150 minutes of moderate aerobic exercise per week, or 75 minutes of weekly aerobic exercise, is relatively well known (Eckel et al., 2014). Most research on physical health has been done on aerobic exercise, but relatively little is known on the effects of other forms of exercise on chronic medical condition. The literature is even more limited for mental disorders. Current understanding on the impact of physical activity on brain function is also largely based on aerobic exercise and its associated physiological effects.

In contrast, it is not unusual to find people with psychological distress seeking alternative interventions to reduce distress. These interventions frequently include an element of physical activity, but they are not exclusively based on aerobics. Although they have their origins in spiritual pursuits in ancient times, yoga, tai chi and meditation have been common practices in Asian communities for enhancing health and stress management. This group of exercises is generally conceptualized as mind-body exercise, with core elements of breathing, coordinated movements and meditation. Mind-body exercise frequently entails conscious deliberation to enhance self-awareness and understanding of subtle body sensations. Recent studies have added an empirical dimension for the potential effectiveness of mind-body exercise in symptom alleviation of different psychosomatic conditions and mental disorders.

In Chapter 9, Varambally and Gangadhar have conducted a comprehensive review of clinical studies of yoga on different mental disorders. Starting with a brief introduction of the spiritual roots and practice framework of classical yoga, they review the current evidence on yoga interventions from a therapeutic perspective. There appears to be evidence to suggest that yoga interventions are potentially effective in alleviating symptoms of depression and anxiety. It is interesting to note that selected practice of yoga may possibly be helpful for cognitive and mood symptoms associated with schizophrenia, but the authors caution that meditative practice in yoga may not be advisable in susceptible individuals. Apart from yoga, other mind-body practices should also be explored for more definitive evidence as a potential treatment modality for mental disorders. Mindfulness-based cognitive therapies (psychosocial interventions emphasizing the practice of meditation with coordinated movements) have gained popularity and are showing evidence for the treatment of major depressive disorder that is comparable to medication.

Neuroscience research is starting to suggest that physical activities influence brain function and alter physiological status and neuroplastic response. Research offers theoretical support to the empirical evidence that exercise interventions are important adjuvant approaches in the management of mental disorders. The authors in this book, apart from highlighting updated reviews of the subject, also provide guidelines on how to engage patients in exercise practices, along with tips on sustained practice and adherence. As interest and experience increase, we anticipate that health professionals and medical practitioners will find these tips immensely helpful in their daily practice.

References

Eckel RH, Jakicic JM, Ard JD, de Jesus JM, Houston Miller N, Hubbard VS, Lee IM, Lichtenstein AH, Loria CM, Millen BE, Nonas CA, Sacks FM, Smith SC Jr, Svetkey LP, Wadden TA, Yanovski SZ. American College of Cardiology/American Heart Association Task Force on Practice Guidelines. 2014. 2013 AHA/ACC guideline on lifestyle management to reduce cardiovascular risk: a report of the American College of Cardiology/American Heart Association Task Force on Practice Guidelines. *J Am Coll Cardiol*, 63(25 Pt B), 2960–84.

Kessler RC, Chiu WT, Demler O, Merikangas KR, Walters EE. 2005. Prevalence, severity, and comorbidity of 12-month DSM-IV disorders in the National Comorbidity Survey Replication. *Arch Gen Psychiatry*, 62, 617–27.

Schizophrenia Working Group of the Psychiatric Genomics Consortium. 2014, 24 July. Biological insights from 108 schizophrenia-associated genetic loci. *Nature*, 511, 421–7.

Whiteford HA, Ferrari AJ, Degenhardt L, Feigin V, Vos T. 2015. The global burden of mental, neurological and substance use disorders: an analysis from the Global Burden of Disease Study 2010. *PLoS One*, 10, e0116820.

2

Exercise interventions for youth with psychiatric disorders

Richard R. Dopp

This chapter discusses clinical research on the use of exercise to influence neurodevelopment and serve as treatment for depression, with a focus on youth with autism spectrum disorders (ASD) or depressive disorders. The chapter begins with a discussion of critical developmental periods, highlighting changes within the brain and body that have an impact on the onset of psychiatric symptoms and the response to exercise interventions. The section on neuro-developmental disorders describes motor deficits, coordination disorders, sleep problems, and obesity among youth with ASD, as well as exercise intervention research targeting these difficulties. The section on depressive disorders discusses decreases in physical activity, coupled with increases in depression, that occur during adolescence, and the role of exercise as treatment for adolescents with depressive disorders.

Developmental changes relevant to exercise behavior

Brain, neuromuscular, and cardiovascular development are shaped by the inter-actions of environment, genetic predispositions, and physiological abilities. Prenatal brain development occurs through specific sequences and embryologic processes including neuronal proliferation, migration, differentiation, and early stages of maturation (Barkovich, 1998). Magnetic resonance imaging (MRI) and autopsy studies in infants show dramatic changes in the development of the central nervous system during the first two years of life, with clear evidence of increased myelination and maturation (Ednick, 2009; Kinney, 2005). Yiallourou and colleagues describe a shift in control of the cardiovascular system in infancy from sympathetic to parasympathetic dominance over heart rate and blood pressure (Yiallourou, 2012). The development of physical movement in the first

Physical Exercise Interventions for Mental Health, ed. Linda C. W. Lam and Michelle Riba. Published by Cambridge University Press. © Cambridge University Press 2016.

year of life occurs first at a kinematic level through repetition and practice, followed by changes in nervous and muscular systems (Teulier, 2012). Patterns of physical activity and sleep are not predetermined at birth. Newborn infants typically sleep 16–17 hours per day with significant changes in rest-activity cycles during the first year of life; these changes result in average sleep periods of 8–9 hours by age one (Anders, 1985).

Childhood and adolescence are critical periods in brain development, with peak synaptic density occurring during childhood (Rakic, 1994). Giedd and colleagues examined brain development by conducting repeated brain MRI scans on healthy boys and girls, demonstrating linear increases in white matter; nonlinear changes in cortical gray matter were also observed with evidence of a preadolescent increase followed by a postadolescent decrease (Giedd, 1999). Wu and colleagues examined 133 healthy subjects aged 10–18 years, using diffusion tensor imaging (DTI), identifying evidence of increased myelination in the sensorimotor and temporoparietel regions as well as varied patterns of superficial white matter and gray matter changes, depending on the need for that region to integrate information using multiple sensory modalities (Wu, 2014).

One conceptual model that has been proposed to account for the onset of numerous psychiatric disorders during adolescence suggests that illness may develop when there is a problem with brain reorganization or "moving parts get broken" (Paus, 2008). Problems with brain reorganization may allow for the development of ASD in young children as well as the development of depression during adolescence. At the same time, the activities and experiences in which youth engage will help determine the trajectory of their physical, social, and emotional growth. It is this perspective that generates interest in physical activity and exercise interventions for children with ASDs and for adolescents with depression; exercise can have a positive impact on brain development during these critical life stages and can specifically address the clinical symptoms present in these disorders.

Neurodevelopmental disorders

In the 1960s, epidemiological estimates of the prevalence of autism were at 0.7%, or 1 in 143 (Treffert, 1970). The Centers for Disease Control website stated that the CDC's Autism and Developmental Disabilities Monitoring Network reported 1 in 88 children were identified with ASD in 2013, and by 2014 that prevalence had increased to 1 in 68 (CDC, 2014). National Health Statistics Reports describe a significant rise in the prevalence of parent-reported ASD diagnoses over a recent five-year period, from 1.16% (1 in 86) in 2007 to 2% (1 in 50) in 2012 (Blumberg, 2013). The causes of autism spectrum disorders are multifactorial involving both genetic predispositions and environmental contributions (Tordjman, 2014). One recent review highlighted the role of perinatal stress or maternal infection during pregnancy that triggers pro-inflammatory and neurotoxic molecules that cross the blood-brain barrier, interfering with normal brain development and causing some cases of ASDs (Angelidou, 2012). More recently, the American Academy of Psychiatry revised the classification of ASDs in the *Diagnostic and Statistical Manual*, 5th edition (DSM-5), incorporating several diagnoses, which were previously included individually in DSM-IV: autistic disorder, Asperger's disorder, childhood disintegrative disorder, and pervasive development disorder not otherwise specified (PDD NOS) (APA, 2013). These previously discrete diagnoses have always shared characteristics of impaired social communication and restricted interests, but have only recently been combined under one set of diagnostic criteria. These changes in diagnostic classification will need to be considered in future prevalence estimates for ASD. However, the increasing prevalence of ASD was observed well before modification of diagnostic categories took place.

Along with impairment in social communication and restrictions in behaviors, interests, and activities, motor deficits are pervasive across ASDs and are considered by some to be cardinal features of the diagnosis (Landa & Garrett-Meyer, 2006). Reduced levels of motor coordination have been observed in youth diagnosed with either autistic disorder or Asperger's disorder, with early reports of less impairment in the Asperger's disorder group (Ghaziuddin, 1994). Follow-up studies comparing motor coordination for youth with autistic disorder, Asperger's disorder, and pervasive developmental disorder showed no between-group differences in coordination once the intellectual quotient was included in the model; lower levels of intelligence in some youth with autistic disorder may account for aspects of impairment observed on tests of motor coordination (Ghaziuddin & Butler, 1998).

Many youth who meet criteria for an ASD diagnosis also will meet criteria for developmental coordination disorder (Miyahara, 2013), with a range of functional challenges in fine motor control and more complex movement, such as walking and running. In a study of 159 young children, 136 with ASD and 23 without the diagnosis, significant correlations were seen in measures of gross and fine motor skills, and scores of calibrated autism severity, with impairment in motor skills predicting deficits in social communication (MacDonald, 2014). Iosa and colleagues used triaxial accelerometry to measure trunk movements and stability for seven youth with Down syndrome, four with autistic disorder, seven with PDD NOS, and a control group of seven typically developing youth. Participants were measured during trials of walking, running, and running with a soccer ball at their feet (dribbling). There were no differences between the participants with intellectual disabilities and the control group during walking, but speed differences emerged during running tasks with healthy participants demonstrating greater speed and stability along the craniocaudal axis. During the dribbling task, the participants with autistic disorder demonstrated greater instability in the anteroposterior and laterolateral axes as well (Iosa, 2014). The potential for loss of balance or the level of coordination deficit may increase as tasks become more complex, such as those required when participating in sports.

Sleep problems and obesity also are commonly reported among youth with ASDs. Studies comparing sleep for youth with ASDs to that of healthy controls demonstrate significantly more difficulty with initiation of sleep and significantly more daytime sleepiness in children with ASDs (Bruni, 2007). Souders and colleagues compared 59 children with ASDs to 40 typically developing controls using the Children's Sleep Habits Questionnaire (Owens, 2000), a scored 33-item parent report that evaluates sleep behavior within eight different subscales: bedtime resistance, sleep-onset delay, sleep duration, sleep anxiety, night wakings, parasomnias, sleep-disordered breathing, and daytime sleepiness. Elevated levels of sleep disturbance in the ASD cohort were reported by 66% of parents compared with 45% in the typically developing cohort (Souders, 2009). This not only supports previous research demonstrating very high rates of sleep disturbance in children with ASD (Elrod & Hood, 2015), but also adds to the evidence of sleep disturbance for youth in the general population (Reiter & Rosen, 2014). With respect to obesity, in a sample of youth obtained from the National Survey of Children's Health, the prevalence of obesity in children with ASDs was 30.4% compared with a prevalence of 23.6% in age-matched children without ASDs (Curtin, 2010). A retrospective chart review of 273 children with ASD found that 39% of those with autistic disorder had a body mass index (BMI) in the overweight or obese range (Egan, 2013). Compounding the problem, atypical antipsychotics (AAPs) are frequently used with children and adolescents (Olfson, 2006), including those with ASD. Evidence supports the use of antipsychotic medication for aggressive behavior and AAPs are considered safer than traditional antipsychotic medications. However, there are still important risks with these medications including significant weight gain resulting in metabolic syndrome, diabetes, sleep apnea, stroke, blood clots, and even sudden cardiac death (Allison, 1999). For children and teens with both ASD and obesity, psychosocial challenges can be exacerbated, resulting in comorbid anxiety or depression. Additional medications such as metformin have shown some effectiveness in controlling weight gain (Klein, 2006), but often have limited advantages due to compliance issues.

Recognizing that motor issues, sleep problems, and obesity are major issues for youth with ASD has led to a call for exercise interventions that can address these difficulties. In seeking to develop and assess such programs, researchers certainly recognize that changing patterns in an individual and family can be challenging, especially for children with behavior problems. A lack of interest, developmentally appropriate programs, and caregiver time have been identified as barriers to participation in exercise for youth with ASD (Yazdani, 2013). Nevertheless, despite these identified barriers, there is evidence that increased physical activity can be achieved. In families in which the caregivers exercise more than three hours per week, youth with special needs were 4.2 times more likely to be physically active compared with children whose parents were less physically active (Yazdani, 2013). Experimental research designs have demonstrated that children with moderate to severe intellectual disability are capable of increasing their treadmill walking duration. Vashdi and colleagues found that children with intellectual disabilities had fewer attempts to discontinue walking on a treadmill when they had another child walking at the same time (paired modeling) and when positive reinforcement was used by the supervisor or study staff (Vashdi, 2008).

In addition to establishing the feasibility of exercise for children with ASD, research has shown promising outcomes as a result of participation. Exercise interventions for this population have demonstrated a reduction in stereotypic behaviors (Petrus, 2008) and an increase in academic engagement following antecedent exercise (Neely, 2015). One unique study examined the use of video-games to enhance exercise for youth with ASDs, specifically Dance Dance Revolution (DDR) and cyber cycling, which includes a recumbent exercise bike interconnected with a videogame that requires pedaling and steering to chase floating coins and dragons (Anderson-Hanley, 2011). Comparison was made between levels of autistic behavior during a baseline video-watching control session and an exergaming session one week later. Parent/guardians completed the Gilliam Autism Rating Scale, 2nd edition (Gilliam, 2006), which included review of videotapes at each time-point to quantify repetitive behaviors. Improvements were seen after one session of exergaming, compared with the control condition with a reduction in repetitive behaviors and improvement on the Digit Span Backwards test of executive function (Anderson-Hanley, 2011). Hilton and colleagues conducted a 30-session pilot study using the Makato Arena, a martial arts arcade-style training game that challenges participants to move in response to light and sound cues. Although this pilot study did not include a comparison condition, they observed improvements in both motor and executive functioning (Hilton, 2014). Chan and colleagues examined outcomes for 46 children with ASD that were randomly assigned to four weeks of a traditional Chinese mind-body exercise (Nei Yang Gong) or four weeks of progressive muscle relaxation. When compared with participants in the muscle relaxation condition, those randomly assigned to the mind-body exercise demonstrated significantly greater improvement in self-control and parental report of decreased autistic symptoms (Chan, 2013). In a separate study examining the effects of a group swimming program for youth with ASDs, using a within-subjects crossover design, Pan reported significant improvements in aquatic skills, academic behavior, and social behaviors (Pan, 2010). This study by Pan was included in a meta-analysis of 16 studies including 133 children and adults, showing that individuals with ASD who participate in exercise interventions show significant improvement in both physical and psychosocial domains whether that intervention was individual or group (Sowa & Meulenbroek, 2012).

While there are numerous published reports of exercise in youth with ASD, few studies have targeted weight reduction as an outcome. Pitetti and colleagues did examine the effects of a 9-month treadmill walking program for youth with autistic disorder within a school treatment program. They observed an increase in caloric expenditure and a decrease in BMI in the group of children with developmental disabilities who participated in the treadmill walking program compared with a control group that was not part of the treadmill walking program, but did continue to participate in the standard physical education curriculum (Pitetti, 2007). In a different study, Hinckson and colleagues examined the effects of a family-centered weight-management program of shorter duration (10 weeks) that included physical activity and nutrition counseling for individuals with disabilities and their families, demonstrating positive changes in lifestyle habits, but no significant improvements in body composition or BMI (Hinckson, 2013). More research in this area is needed to disentangle the beneficial effects of the exercise itself from the effects of social interactions related to the exercise intervention, a "social confound" that exists in exercise research. Weight and BMI may be outcome variables that are more likely to be influenced by the effects of the exercise than by the effects of the social interaction. Improvements in psychosocial functioning may be influenced both by the physiological impact of exercise and the social interactions of the intervention.

Depressive disorders

Depression exists in young children, latency-age children, and adolescents, with prevalence of depressive disorders increasing significantly during adolescence. Evidence suggests significant sex differences in the emergence of this disease. Longitudinal studies show that while males and females have similar rates of depression until age twelve, the rate of depression in females is nearly double that for males by late adolescence (Hankin, 1998), approaching levels consistent with adult female populations (Lewinsohn, 1998). The onset of depression during the critical developmental period of adolescence is a growing public health concern, as it is associated with impairment in psychosocial and academic functioning, and predicts recurrent episodes of major depression in adulthood (Lewinsohn, 2003).

In considering behavioral patterns that may play a role in depression, there is a growing interest in physical activity. Physical activity is declining for youth in many countries around the world as a result of increased sedentary use of electronics, changes in transportation, decreases in physical education in school, and declining rates of participation in sports (Dollman, 2005). Data from the Youth Risk Behavior Survey suggests that physical activity levels decrease steadily throughout high school years, with females more likely than males to be insufficiently active (less than 30 minutes at least three times per week) at all grade levels (Grunbaum, 2002).

These age and sex patterns raise questions regarding the relationship between physical activity and depression in adolescents. Motl and colleagues reported data from a sample of more than 4,500 adolescents in the United States at three time points during their seventh and eighth grade years. Naturally occurring changes in physical activity were negatively correlated with changes in depressive symptoms on the Center for Epidemiological Studies Depression Scale (Motl, 2004). In other words, youth who reported an increase in physical activity outside of school also reported a decrease in depressive symptoms. Another study reported data from 736 adolescents in the United Kingdom, assessing physical activity through the measurement of heart rate and movement sensing in early adolescence (initial assessment mean age 14.5 years) and depressive symptoms in later adolescence, approximately three years later (Goodyer, 2009; Toseeb, 2014). The investigators found that the level of physical activity in early adolescence did not predict levels of depressive symptoms or diagnoses of major depressive disorders three years later and suggested that the effect of physical activity on depressed mood may be small or nonexistent among adolescents (Toseeb, 2014). There are several possible explanations for the failure of physical activity level to predict an assessment of depressive symptoms. As previously described, the risk for depression is greatest among adolescent females, and a previous article of this same dataset reported that 81% of the female adolescents were inactive (Corder, 2011). Also, this sample of adolescents was engaged in mostly light intensity physical activity (517 minutes per day) and sedentary time (364 minutes per day), with low levels of moderate physical activity (38 minutes per day) and very low levels of vigorous activity (3.4 minutes per day) (Collings, 2014).

Few studies have examined the effects of an exercise intervention for youth with clinically significant depressive disorders, and even fewer include higher levels of aerobic exercise, which have been shown to be more effective at reducing depressive symptoms (Dunn, 2005; Hughes, 2013). In their study examining the efficacy of exercise as treatment for depression in adults, Dunn and colleagues randomly assigned participants to one of five treatment conditions that varied by intensity (high-dose exercise, low-dose exercise, stretching-control) and frequency (three or five times per week). In this 12-week exercise intervention, all sessions were conducted individually in a structured, supervised setting. An intent-to-treat analysis of participants' scores on the 17-item Hamilton Depression Rating Scale (Hamilton, 1960) showed a reduction of 47% for participants in the public health dose exercise condition compared with 30% for the participants in the low-dose exercise condition and 29% for those in the stretching-control condition (Dunn, 2005).

A randomized controlled trial of older adults with depression compared supervised exercise, home-based exercise, sertraline, and pill placebo (Blumenthal, 2007). Participants in the supervised exercise condition attended three group exercise sessions per week for 16 weeks. Each aerobic exercise session began with a 10-minute warm-up walk on a treadmill followed by 30 minutes of walking or jogging at an intensity that would keep their heart rate within the assigned range (70% to 85% maximum heart rate reserve as measured by graded treadmill exercise testing). Participants in the home-based exercise program were given similar exercise prescriptions based upon their treadmill testing with minimal contact with study staff. Participants in the pill conditions were provided with sertraline or matching placebo by the treating psychiatrist. Sertraline dosing was started at 50 mg with subsequent increases by 50 mg up to 200 mg daily depending upon response and side effects. Depression severity was measured using the Hamilton Depression Rating Scale at baseline and 16 weeks. Rates of remission across the four groups were as follows: supervised exercise (46%), home-based exercise (38%), medication (44%), and placebo control (26%).

These results represent intent-to-treat analyses, but there was a higher dropout rate reported for the supervised exercise condition (20%) than for home-based exercise (6%) or sertraline (7%). Additionally, the supervised and home-based exercisers had similar rates of compliance, but the supervised exercisers tended to push themselves into their target heart rate range more consistently (Blumenthal, 2007). Data from the one-year follow-up assessment showed that rates of Major Depressive Disorder (MDD) remission continued to rise to 66% for all participants and that self-report rates of exercise during the follow-up period predicted both Hamilton Depression Rating Scale scores and MDD diagnosis (Hoffman, 2011).

The evidence for exercise in depressed adults is impressive, but there are concerns about whether teenagers with depression would be willing to participate in such programs. Informed by these interventions in adults with depression, Dopp and colleagues conducted a study to examine the feasibility of an exercise intervention for youth with clinically significant depressive disorders. The study design included a mix of supervised and home-based exercise sessions with three supervised exercise sessions in the first week, two in the second week, and one in weeks 3 through 12. Participants were expected to complete one independent exercise session in week 2 and two in weeks 3 through 12. Adolescent assent and parental consent were obtained from 14 adolescents. One participant sustained a major orthopedic injury prior to initiating the exercise intervention. Thirteen participants (female = 9), with a mean age of 15.2 (SD = 1.4) years, initiated the intervention phase of the study. Eleven participants met criteria for Major Depressive Disorder and two for Depressive Disorder Not Otherwise Specified. At baseline, 9 of the 13 participants were in psychotherapy and/or medication treatment for their depression. Seven participants were taking no psychotropic medications during the study. Five participants were on selective serotonin reuptake inhibitors (SSRIs) at the beginning of the intervention (four on fluoxetine and one on sertraline) and continued on them throughout the intervention. Three of the five participants on SSRIs at baseline were also taking stimulants. During the intervention, two participants initiated psychotherapy, and one participant began taking an SSRI (sertraline) at approximately the three-week time-point. During the intervention, two unmedicated participants terminated their psychotherapy treatment for depression, both citing an improvement in mood as the reason for termination.

All participants completed the 15 supervised exercise sessions and 21 independent exercise sessions. Actigraphy recordings in weeks 3 and 12 were used to verify the independent exercise sessions, verifying 81% compliance with expected independent exercise sessions during those two weeks. Heart rate goals (220 – age X 0.85) were established and participants hit their targets in 79% of the supervised exercise sessions. Participants with higher average heart rates, recorded during the supervised exercise sessions, showed greater reductions in BMI. Depression was measured via semistructured interviews using the Children's Depression Rating Scale- Revised (CDRS-R) (Poznanski & Mokros, 1996). The mean score on the CDRS-R for these 13 participants was

48.9 (SD = 9.7) at baseline and 28.5 (SD = 10.4) post-intervention. Remission of depression, as defined by a CDRS-R score < 28, was achieved by 62% of participants at the conclusion of the 12-week intervention. The results of this study showed that research investigating exercise as treatment for depression in adolescents is feasible, but definitive conclusions regarding the specific effects of exercise on depression cannot be made in the absence of a control condition (Dopp, 2012).

In the Depressed Adolescents Treated with Exercise (DATE) study, Hughes and colleagues randomly assigned untreated adolescents meeting criteria for major depressive disorder to either vigorous exercise or a control-stretching condition for 12 weeks. Accelerometry was used to measure activity levels throughout the study with a target of >12 kcal/kg/week for those in the exercise condition and a target of <4 kcal/kg/week for those in the stretching control condition. The protocol included three supervised physical activity sessions in the first two weeks of the study, followed by one supervised session in weeks 3 through 12, during which time participants completed their two independent exercise sessions at home or other locations. The amount of time spent participating in supervised physical activity was the same for both groups, with the only difference being the amount of energy expended during the activity. Participants in both groups demonstrated significant increases in physical activity and significant decreases in depressive symptoms. At week 12, the participants in the exercise condition had a 100% response rate (86% remission), while participants in the stretching control group had a 67% response rate (50% remission). Hughes and colleagues concluded that exercise interventions have promise as a nonmedication treatment for depression in adolescents and that further randomized controlled trials are merited (Hughes, 2013).

Considering results from research that includes combination treatment with antidepressant medication and therapy is useful in assessing this conclusion. One of the best known randomized controlled trials in adolescent depression is the Treatment for Adolescents with Depression Study (TADS), which compared the effectiveness of four treatments: fluoxetine, cognitive behavioral therapy (CBT), combination with fluoxetine and CBT, and pill placebo (March, 2004). The inclusion criteria for TADS were youth aged 12–17 years who met DSM-IV diagnosis of MDD and scored 45 or above on the CDRS-R at baseline. Adolescents with higher levels of dangerous behavior, such as recent hospitalization, suicide attempt in the last six months, or elevated suicidal ideation in the context of a disorganized family unable to guarantee safety monitoring, were excluded. Rates of response for fluoxetine with CBT were 71%, for fluoxetine alone 61%, CBT alone 43%, and placebo 35%. Based in part on these results, the combination of medication and evidence-based psychotherapy such as CBT has been considered the standard of treatment for adolescents with depression (March & Vitiello, 2009).

In the Treatment of Resistant Depression in Adolescents (TORDIA) study, treatment options were examined for youth who were nonresponders to initial attempts at treatment with a selective serotonin reuptake inhibitor (SSRI) such as fluoxetine or paroxetine (Brent, 2008). Adolescents with depression were randomly assigned to one of four treatment groups for 12 weeks; (1) different SSRI, (2) different SSRI and CBT, (3) venlafaxine, or (4) venlafaxine and CBT. The response rates were higher for CBT and a switch to a different medication (54.8%) than a medication switch alone (40.5%). There was no significant difference in response rate between venlafaxine (48.2%) and a second SSRI (47.0%). While the TADS study excluded individuals with clinically significant suicidal ideation due to concerns of randomization to 12 weeks of no treatment in the placebo condition, TORDIA consisted of four active treatment arms and included individuals with more chronic depression and higher levels of suicidal ideation. In their 24-week outcomes article, Emslie and colleagues suggest that the lower rates of remission in TORDIA when compared with TADS may be due to these differences in the study sample, which have been shown to predict lower levels of response to treatment (Emslie, 2010). Similar to the results of most studies in depression, the combination of medication and therapy was found to be more effective than either modality used alone.

Thus, it is important to note that the response and remission rates reported for the exercise intervention in the DATE study by Hughes and colleagues exceeded those demonstrated for the combination of medication and therapy received in TADS and TORDIA. Nevertheless, adolescents with severe suicidal ideation, previous history of suicide attempt, or severe depression (CDRS-R>70) were excluded from DATE, and the response rate in the stretching-control group was quite high, leaving questions unanswered regarding how to best include youth with more severe depression and what represents appropriate control conditions. To further explore these issues, Dopp and colleagues randomly assigned 18 adolescents with clinically significant depressive symptoms (CDRS-R >40), and low levels of physical activity, to an exercise intervention or a treatment-as-usual comparison condition. Participants in both conditions were allowed to continue their current treatment as long as that treatment was stable (i.e., those on antidepressants had been on a stable dose for at least 4 weeks). Reductions in CDRS-R scores were significantly greater for participants in the exercise intervention compared with those in the treatment-as-usual condition, further supporting the use of exercise as a stand-alone or combination treatment for youth with depression (unpublished data). The benefits of this research design, with both an exercise intervention and a treatment-as-usual comparison condition, allowed for the inclusion of adolescents with higher levels of depression and suicidality as well as the ability to control for the number of contacts with study staff. The exercise sessions were conducted individually, which prevented confounding by social interaction among the adolescents. At the same time, interventions that involve only individual exercise sessions are more labor-intensive and limit the availability of supported exercise to fewer numbers of adolescents.

In a study examining the effects of group exercise for adolescent females with depression, Nabkasorn and colleagues used a crossover design that randomly assigned participants to an 8-week jogging group (5 days per week for 50 minutes) or to 8 weeks of usual daily activities. At the 8-week time-point, participants who had been in the running group were expected to resume their previous level of activity, while those in the initial usual activity condition were enrolled in their own 8-week running group. There were significant reductions in the level of depression for those participants who initiated in the running group compared with those randomized to usual daily activity. As the authors described their results, they commented on 5 participants from the initial running group who were excluded from their analyses at the 16-week time-point because they were unable to "maintain the usual level of physical activity constant in their non-exercising period" (Nabkasorn, 2006, p. 180). In other words, these participants refused to stop exercising. This is consistent with other published data for adolescents with depression, which demonstrated the maintenance of elevated levels of physical activity following the conclusion of the initial period of supported exercise (Dopp, 2012). It provides evidence for the extent to which physical activity regimens are acceptable to this population, creating opportunities for long-term positive outcomes.

Conclusion

Humans are meant to move. Our brains and bodies develop, grow, and mature in response to our physical activities, behaviors, and experiences. For children and adolescents with psychiatric disorders such as ASD and depression, the importance of physical activity and exercise cannot be overstated. The course of illness in both ASD and depression can be positively influenced through engagement in exercise, with physical activity serving as the experiential prompt that moves brain development in a positive direction. Similar to the way in which playing the piano has been found to have a positive impact on the fiber tract organization of the brain in children, adolescents, and adults (Bengtsson, 2005), exercise may play a crucial role in brain reorganization especially during periods of early childhood and adolescence. The strong relationships among mental health, physical health, sleep, and obesity support the need for exercise for all youth.

The social communication deficits seen in ASD are correlated with motor deficits, suggesting that improvements in the area of physical activity may facilitate improvements in social behaviors (Sowa & Meulenbroek, 2012). Exercise that precedes educational sessions is associated with a reduction in stereotypic behavior and an increase in eye contact with teachers (Neely, 2015), enhancing learning opportunities for students with ASD. Physical activity and exercise have significant effects on sleep and metabolism, with potential to address the problems with sleep and weight that are pervasive in the general population and in youth with psychiatric disorders.

Although no large-scale effectiveness studies have yet been conducted looking at exercise as treatment for depression in adolescents, numerous studies have demonstrated the feasibility of exercise as treatment for this vulnerable population. For adolescents with depression, exercise interventions have shown significant reductions in symptom severity, even among patients who had not responded to standard treatments. The reductions in depressive symptoms observed in these studies are comparable and often greater than the reductions seen in research studies using gold-standard treatments of evidence-based psychotherapies combined with antidepressant medications.

However, despite these robust findings, it is clear that many published studies in the medical literature are limited by the absence of control groups or between-subject designs, small sample sizes, and a shortage of long-term outcomes (Srinivasan, 2014). More research is needed. The most effective strategies for engaging youth in exercise behaviors should be identified, and exercise programs fine-tuned for youth populations with varying symptoms. Questions related to appropriate control or comparison conditions in exercise research should be answered, taking into account safety concerns for youth with depression and suicidal ideation. Ethical questions arise when at-risk youth are randomized to control conditions that delay treatment. Introducing exercise along with other treatments may be one approach; add-on studies of exercise have shown significant reductions in depression severity, while allowing participants to continue in other forms of treatment with medication and psychotherapy (Dopp, 2012). Investigators need to develop and assess group strategies that can increase the reach of exercise programs among youth with mental health problems. The role of exercise to treat adults with ASD or depression also should be explored. These and other issues remain on a research agenda that is increasingly urgent in light of prevalence trends regarding ASD, depression, and other psychiatric disorders among young people and adults.

Although unanswered questions remain, presently available evidence underscores the feasibility, acceptability, and benefits of exercise for youth with psychiatric disorders. Now is the time for physicians and mental health professionals of all disciplines to give careful consideration to the inclusion of exercise as part of the treatment plan for their patients with autism spectrum disorders (Lochbaum, 1995) and depression. The medical profession should identify strategies to translate exercise research findings into clinical practice, provide guidance to physicians and other healthcare providers in the implementation of evidence-based physical activity interventions, and integrate exercise programs into our systems of healthcare delivery, especially for youth with psychiatric disorders.

References

Allison, D.B., Mentore, J.L., Heo, M., et al. (1999). Antipsychotic-induced weight gain: a comprehensive research synthesis. *American Journal of Psychiatry*, 156(11),1686–1696.

American Psychiatric Association. (2013). *Diagnostic and statistical manual of mental disorders, fifth edition, DSM-5*. Washington D.C.: American Psychiatric Publishing.

Anders, T.F., Keener, M.A., Kraemer, H. (1985). Sleep-wake state organization, neonatal assessment and development in premature infants during the first year of life. *Sleep*, 8(3),193–206.

Anderson-Hanley, C., Tureck, K., Schneiderman, R.L. (2011). Autism and exergaming: effects on repetitive behaviors and cognition. *Psychology Research and Behavior Management*, 4. 129–137.

Angelidou, A., Asadi, S., Alysandratos, K.D., et al. (2012). Perinatal stress, brain inflammation and risk of autism-review and proposal. *Biomed Central Pediatrics*, 12(89),1–12.

Barkovich, A.J. (1998). MR of the normal neonatal brain: assessment of deep structures. *American Journal of Neuroradiology*, 19, 1397–1403.

Bengtsson, S.L., Nagy, Z., Skare, S., et al. (2005). Extensive piano practicing has regionally specific effects on white matter development. *Nature Neuroscience*, 8(9),1148–1150.

Blumberg, S.J., Bramlett, M.D., Kogan, M.D., et al. (2013). Changes in prevalence of parent-reported autism spectrum disorder in school-aged U.S. children: 2007 to 2011–2012. *National Health Statistics Report*, 20(65),1–11.

Blumenthal, J.A., Babyak, M.A., Doraiswamy, P.M., et al. (2007). Exercise and pharmacotherapy in the treatment of major depressive disorder. *Psychosomatic Medicine*, 69(7),587–596.

Brent, D., Emslie, G., Clarke, G., et al. (2008). Switching to another SSRI or to venlafaxine with or without cognitive behavioral therapy for adolescents with SSRI-resistant depression: the TORDIA randomized controlled trial. *JAMA*, 299(8),901–913.

Bruni, O., Ferri, R., Vittori, E., et al. (2007). Sleep architecture and NREM alterations in children and adolescents with Asperger syndrome. *Sleep*, 30, 1577–1585.

Centers for Disease Control and Prevention. (2014). Prevalence of autism spectrum disorder among children aged 8 years—autism and developmental disabilities monitoring network. *Morbidity and Mortality Weekly Report Surveillance Summaries*, 63(2),1–21.

Chan, A.S., Sze, S.L., Siu, N.Y., et al. (2013). A Chinese mind-body exercise improves self-control of children with autism: a randomized controlled trial. *PLOS ONE*, 8(7),1–12.

Collings, P.J., Wijndaele, K., Corder, K., et al. (2014). Levels and patterns of objectively-measured physical activity volume and intensity distribution in UK adolescents: the ROOTS study. *International Journal of Behavioral Nutrition and Physical Activity*, 11(23),1–12.

Corder, K., van Sluijs, E.M., Goodyer, I., et al. (2011). Physical activity awareness of British adolescents. *Archives of Pediatric & Adolescent Medicine*, 165(7), 603–609.

Curtin, C., Anderson, S.E., Must, A., Bandini, L. (2010). The prevalence of obesity in children with autism: a secondary data analysis using nationally representative data from the National Survey of Children's Health. *Biomed Central Pediatrics*, 10(11),1–5.

Dollman, J., Norton, K., Norton, L. (2005). Evidence for secular trends in children's physical activity behavior. *British Journal of Sports Medicine*, 39(12),892–897.

Dopp, R.R., Mooney, A.J., Armitage, R., King, C. (2012). Exercise for adolescents with depressive disorders: a feasibility study. *Depression Research and Treatment*. Available from: http://www.ncbi.nlm.nih.gov/pmc/articles/PMC3409521/pdf/DRT2012-257472.pdf/ [24 July 2012]

Dunn, A.L., Trivedi, M.H., Kampert, J.B., et al. (2005). Exercise treatment for depression: efficacy and dose response. *American Journal of Preventive Medicine*, 28(1),1–8.

Ednick, M., Cohen, A.P., McPhail, G.L., et al. (2009). A review of the effects of sleep during the first year of life on cognitive, psychomotor, and temperament development. *Sleep*, 32(11),1449–1458.

Egan, A.M., Dreyer, M.L., Odar, C.C., et al. (2013). Obesity in young children with autism spectrum disorders: prevalence and associated factors. *Childhood Obesity*, 9(2),125–131.

Elrod, M.G., Hood, B.S. (2015). Sleep differences among children with autism spectrum disorders and typically developing peers: a meta-analysis. *Journal of Developmental and Behavioral Pediatrics*, 36(3),166–177.

Emslie, G.J., Mayes, T., Porta, G., et al. (2010). Treatment of Resistant Depression in Adolescents (TORDIA): week 24 outcomes. *American Journal of Psychiatry*, 167(7),782–791.

Ghaziuddin, M., Butler, E. (1998). Clumsiness in autism and Asperger syndrome: a further report. *Journal of Intellectual Disabilities*, 42, 43–48.

Ghaziuddin, M., Butler, E., Tsai, L., Ghaziuddin, N. (1994). Is clumsiness a marker for Asperger syndrome?. *Journal of Intellectual Disabilities*, 38, 519–527.

Giedd, J.N., Blumenthal, J., Jeffries, N.O., et al. (1999). Brain development during childhood and adolescence: a longitudinal MRI study. *Nature Neuroscience*, 2(10),861–863.

Gilliam, J. (2006). *GARS-2: Gilliam Autism Rating Scale*. 2nd edition. Austin, TX. PRO-ED.

Goodyer, I.M., Bacon, A., Ban, M., et al., (2009). Serotonin transporter genotype, morning cortisol and subsequent depression in adolescents. *British Journal of Psychiatry*, 195(1),39–45.

Grunbaum, J.A., Kann, L., Kinchen, S.A., et al. (2002). Youth risk behavior surveillance—United States, 2001. *Journal of School Health*, 72(8),313–328.

Hamilton, M. (1960). A rating scale for depression. *Journal of Neurology, Neurosurgery & Psychiatry*, 23, 56–62.

Hankin, B.L., Abramson, L.Y., Moffitt, T.E., et al. (1998). Development of depression from preadolescence to young adulthood: emerging gender differences in a 10-year longitudinal study. *Journal of Abnormal Psychology*, 107(1),128–140.

Hilton, C.L., Cumpata, K., Klohr, C., et al. (2014). Effects of exergaming on executive function and motor skills in children with autism spectrum disorder: a pilot study. *American Journal of Occupational Therapy*, 68(1),57–65.

Hinckson, E.A., Dickinson, A., Water, T., et al. (2013). Physical activity, dietary habits and overall health in overweight and obese children and youth with intellectual disability or autism. *Research in Development Disabilities*, 34(4),1170–1178.

Hoffman, B.M., Babyak, M.A., Craighead, W.E., et al. (2011). Exercise and pharmacotherapy in patients with major depression: one-year follow-up of the SMILE study. *Psychosomatic Medicine*, 73(2),127–133.

Hughes, C.W., Barnes, S., Barnes, C., et al. (2013). Depressed Adolescents Treated with Exercise (DATE): A pilot randomized controlled trial to test feasibility and establish preliminary effect sizes. *Mental Health and Physical Activity*, 6(2),1–32.

Iosa, M., Morelli, D., Nisi, E., et al. (2014). Assessment of upper body accelerations in young adults with intellectual disabilities while walking, running, and dual-task running. *Human Movement Science*, 34, 187–195.

Kinney, H.C. (2005). Human myelination and perinatal white matter disorders. *Journal of Neurological Sciences*, 228(2),190–192.

Klein, D.J., Cottingham, E.M., Sorter, M., et al. (2006). A randomized, double-blind, placebo-controlled trial of metformin treatment of weight gain associated with initiation of atypical antipsychotic therapy in children and adolescents. *American Journal of Psychiatry*, 163(12),2072–2079.

Landa, R., Garrett-Meyer, E. (2006). Development in infants with autism spectrum disorders: a prospective study. *Journal of Child Psychology and Psychiatry*, 47(6),629–638.

Lewinsohn, P.M., Rohde, P., Seeley, J.R. (1998). Major depressive disorder in older adolescents: prevalence, risk factors, and clinical implications. *Clinical Psychology Review*, 18(7),765–794.

Lewinsohn, P.M., Rohde, P., Seeley, J.R., et al. (2003). Psychosocial functioning of young adults who have experienced and recovered from major depressive disorder during adolescence. *Journal of Abnormal Psychology*, 112(3),353–363.

Lochbaum, M.R., Crews, D.J. (1995). Exercise prescription for autistic populations. *Journal of Autism and Developmental Disorders*, 25(3),335–336.

MacDonald, M., Lord, C., Ulrich, D.A. (2014). Motor skills and calibrated autism severity in young children with autism spectrum disorder. *Adapted Physical Activity Quarterly*, 31(2),95–105.

March, J., Silva, S., Petrycki, S., et al. (2004). Fluoxetine, cognitive-behavioral therapy, and their combination for adolescents with depression: Treatment for Adolescents with Depression Study (TADS) randomized controlled trial. *JAMA*, 292(7),807–820.

March, J.S., Vitiello, B. (2009). Clinical messages from the Treatment for Adolescents with Depression Study (TADS). *American Journal of Psychiatry*, 166(10),1118–1123.

Miyahara, M. (2013). Meta review of systematic and meta analytic reviews on movement differences, effect of movement based interventions, and the underlying neural mechanisms in autism spectrum disorder. *Frontiers in Integrative Neuroscience*, 7(16),1–7.

Motl, R.W., Birnbaum, A.S., Kubik, M.Y., Dishman, R.K. (2004). Naturally occurring changes in physical activity are inversely related to depressive symptoms during early adolescence. *Psychosomatic Medicine*, 66(3),336–342.

Nabkasorn, C., Miyai, N., Sootmongkol, A., et al. (2006). Effects of physical exercise on depression, neuroendocrine stress hormones and physiological fitness in adolescent females with depressive symptoms. *European Journal of Public Health*, 16(2),179–184.

Neely, L., Rispoli, M., Gerow, S., Ninci, J. (2015). Effects of antecedent exercise on academic engagement and stereotypy during instruction. *Behavior Modification*, 39(1),98–116.

Olfson, M., Blanco, C., Liu, L., et al. (2006). National trends in the outpatient treatment of children and adolescents with antipsychotic drugs. *Archives of General Psychiatry*, 63(6),679–685.

Owens, J.A., Spirito, A., McGuinn, M. (2000). The Children's Sleep Habits Questionnaire (CSHQ): psychometric properties of a survey instrument for school-aged children. *Sleep*, 23(8),1043–1051.

Pan, C.Y. (2010). Effects of water exercise swimming program on aquatic skills and social behaviors in children with autism spectrum disorders. *Autism*, 14(1),9–28.

Paus, T., Keshavan, M., Giedd, J.N. (2008). Why do many psychiatric disorders emerge during adolescence? *Nature Reviews Neuroscience*, 9(12),947–957.

Petrus, C., Adamson, S.R., Block, L., Einarson, S.J., et al. (2008). Effects of exercise interventions on stereotypic behaviours in children with autism spectrum disorder. *Physiotherapy Canada*, 60(2),134–145.

Pitetti, K.H., Rendoff, A.D., Grover, T., Beets, M.W. (2007). The efficacy of a 9-month treadmill walking program on the exercise capacity and weight reduction for adolescents with severe autism. *Journal of Autism and Developmental Disorders*, 37(6),997–1006.

Poznanski, E.O., Mokros, H. (1996). *Children's depression rating scale revised (CDRS-R)*. Los Angeles, CA: Western Psychological Services.

Rakic, P., Bourgeois, J.P., Goldman-Rakic, P.S. (1994). Synaptic development of the cerebral cortex: implications for learning, memory, and mental illness. *Progress in Brain Research*, 102, 227–243.

Reiter, J., & Rosen, D. (2014). The diagnosis and management of common sleep disorders in adolescents. *Current Opinions in Pediatrics*, 26(4),407–412.

Souders, M.C., Mason, T.B., Valladares, O., et al. (2009). Sleep behaviors and sleep quality in children with autism spectrum disorders. *Sleep*, 32(12),1566–1578.

Sowa, M., Meulenbroek, R. (2012). Effects of physical exercise on autism spectrum disorders: a meta-analysis. *Research in Autism Spectrum Disorders*, 6, 46–57.

Srinivasan, S.M., Pescatello, L.S., Bhat, A.N. (2014). Current perspectives on physical activity and exercise recommendations for children and adolescents with autism spectrum disorders. *Physical Therapy*, 94(6), 875–889.

Teulier, C., Sansom, J.K., Muraszko, K., Ulrich, B.D. (2012). Longitudinal changes in muscle activity during infants' treadmill stepping. *Journal of Neurophysiology*, 108(3),853–862.

Tordjman, S., Somogyi, E., Coulon, N., et al. (2014). Gene × Environment interactions in autism spectrum disorders: role of epigenetic mechanisms. *Frontiers in Psychiatry*, 5(53),1–17.

Toseeb, U., Brage, S., Corder, K., et al. (2014). Exercise and depressive symptoms in adolescents: a longitudinal cohort study. *JAMA Pediatrics*, 168(12),1093–1100.

Treffert, D.A. (1970). Epidemiology of infantile autism. *Archives of General Psychiatry*, 22(5),431–438.

Vashdi, E., Hutzler, Y., Roth, D. (2008). Compliance of children with moderate to severe intellectual disability to treadmill walking: a pilot study. *Journal of Intellectual Disability Research*, 52, 371–379.

Wu, M., Lu, L.H., Lowes, A., et al. (2014). Development of superficial white matter and its structural interplay with cortical gray matter in children and adolescents. *Human Brain Mapping*, 35, 2806–2816.

Yazdani, S., Yee, C.T., Chung, P.J. (2013). Factors predicting physical activity among children with special needs. *Preventing Chronic Disease*, 10, 1–10.

Yiallourou, S.R., Sands, S.A., Walker, A.M., Horne, R.S. (2012). Maturation of heart rate and blood pressure variability during sleep in term-born infants. *Sleep*, 35(2),177–186.

3

Exercise for the treatment of depression

David A. Baron, Samantha Lasarow and Steven H. Baron

Introduction

The goal of this chapter is to provide an overview and update for clinicians on the role of physical exercise in treating depression, a mental health disorder characterized by low mood, the absence of a positive affect, and a range of emotional, physical, cognitive, and behavioral symptoms. We will provide relevant clinical vignettes, review the extant literature on this topic, and offer treatment recommendations for utilizing exercise as a primary treatment modality and a potential augmentation strategy.

The role of exercise in maintaining physical health and overall fitness has been well documented in the medical literature dating back to ancient times. In the fifth century BC, the Greeks wrote of preserving and restoring health through exercise, and many Greek medical practitioners then and later, such as Herodicus, Hippocrates, and Galen, saw physical well-being as a necessity for mental well-being (Grant, 1991).

Indeed, the positive health effects of regular exercise are well established in the non-psychiatric medical literature. As a popular TV ad in the United States claims, "*Everybody* knows that." However, the role of exercise as a treatment modality for mood disorders is a more recent finding. Exercise has been reported to improve mild cognitive impairment, concentration, focus, and overall mood state. There is no shortage of papers exploring the role of exercise in mood disorders. A Google Scholar search of "Exercise in Treating Depression" resulted in 29,900 hits on October 15, 2014. These papers are the result of clinical observation, clinical trials, and large-scale studies conducted worldwide in a variety of patient populations. The case vignettes offered in this chapter will highlight key clinical issues and relevant take-home points. Of course, no treatment intervention is effective for every patient, and this is

Physical Exercise Interventions for Mental Health, ed. Linda C. W. Lam and Michelle Riba. Published by Cambridge University Press. © Cambridge University Press 2016.

equally true of exercise. However, the low potential adverse side-effect profile of exercise makes it a treatment modality worthy of consideration in virtually every depressed patient. Patients suffering from depression should be under the care of an experienced mental health provider who can monitor symptoms and response to all treatment interventions. Effective treatment strategies should include a bio-psycho-social approach, sensitive to the unique needs of the patient. Not every patient will experience symptom relief from exercise. There are no existing biomarkers that will predict a positive therapeutic response. Exercise has been demonstrated to impact a number of factors related to depression, including brain-derived neurotrophic factor (BDNF), and relief of anxiety. When medically supervised, there are very few adverse side effects associated with this form of treatment. Additional clinical and preclinical research will help determine the optimal utilization of exercise therapy for mood disorders throughout the lifespan.

Treatment interventions for depression

The World Health Organization (WHO) reports that an estimated 350 million people worldwide are affected by depression (Marcus et al., 2012). It is estimated that between 4% and 10% of people worldwide are likely to experience major depression within their lifetimes (Waraich et al., 2004). Numerous treatment interventions for depression have been studied in the literature, ranging from high intensity psychological interventions (e.g., cognitive behavioral therapies [CBT], interpersonal therapy [IPT], behavioral activation, problem solving, short-term psychodynamic psychotherapy, counseling) to pharmacological interventions (antidepressants) and neuromodulation interventions (e.g., light therapy, transcranial magnetic stimulation, electroconvulsive therapy [ECT]) (National Collaborating Centre for Mental Health, 2010).

Depression is a biopsychosocial phenomenon, and, as such, psychosocial factors as well as biological factors must be considered in its treatment. Exercise therapy has measurable biologic effects on a number of organ systems, including the brain, neuroendocrine, pulmonary, cardiac, and musculoskeletal. In addition to its biological effects, exercise can play an important role as a psychosocial intervention. Exercise is maximally effective when it is fun for the patient, and is incorporated into a social activity. As patients engage in an exercise program, self-esteem may be positively impacted as they increase muscle tone, improve sleep, experience an increase in energy levels, improved-self esteem, and feel more in control of their lives. Exercising with friends and loved ones can contribute to enhanced social interactions.

Our first case vignette highlights the role of social supports, using exercise as an adjunct to CBT in treating depression.

A key to success in all treatment modalities is adhering to the prescribed intervention. Medications not taken at the proper dose for the required length of time will not be effective in relieving depressive symptoms; the success of psychotherapy is dependent on the patient making a commitment to attend and engage in the therapy sessions on a regular basis; exercise therapy is no different.

For exercise to be effective in treating the signs and symptoms of depression, the patient must engage in physical activity at least three times per week. This underscores the importance of the exercise program being an enjoyable activity. Patients experiencing adverse side effects from medications tend to be noncompliant. Exercise that is not enjoyable can be compared to adverse side effects resulting from taking an antidepressant, or attempting therapy with a therapist in whom the patient does not have confidence. As with medications and psychotherapy, the "dosing" is important to clinical success. For pharmacotherapy, the proper amount of the medication is critical, as too much will result in adverse side effects and too little will not be efficacious. The appropriate length of psychotherapy is typically determined by the form of therapy employed (some forms of psychotherapy are more focused, with a predetermined number of therapy sessions). Unlike pharmacotherapy and psychotherapy, which tend to be time limited, exercise should become a component of healthy living, and continue even after the depression has resolved. This is a major distinction from the other treatment modalities. Exercise is *both* a treatment modality *and* a healthy life style change to maintain optimal mental *and* physical health.

Case vignette: social exercise as complement to cognitive behavioral therapy

Our first case vignette emphasizes that exercise as a treatment must be prescribed in such a way that patients will be able to adhere to the treatment. Social support has been documented in the literature as an important contributor to adherence to an exercise program (Duncan and McAuley, 1993).

Chief complaint / presenting symptoms: A 44-year-old woman is sent for evaluation of increasingly low mood, loss of libido, poor sleep, and a 20-pound weight gain over the past 6 months.

History of chief complaint: The patient reports gradual onset of her symptoms and cannot recall a triggering event. She is focused on her weight gain and reports this is contributing to her loss of interest in intimacy with her husband. She feels overwhelmed trying to deal with her teenage daughter and reports feeling like a failure as a mother and wife. She tried a fad diet and lost 4 pounds, but has gained back 10 pounds over the past 4 weeks.

Past psych history: Patient reports a bout of depression in her early twenties, but had refused to take medication for fear of weight gain, and was not able to relate to her therapist.

Medical history: Patient is overweight and has mild hypertension. She is in good health otherwise. She gets an annual physical and has no other acute or chronic medical problems.

Family history: She reports her father may have had depression and alcohol abuse, but she is not sure. He was a heavy drinker. She reports no other mental illness in her biological family.

Social history: Patient reports a normal childhood. She denies any history of physical, sexual, or emotional abuse. She got along well with her two siblings, had many friends growing up, and was a good student. She graduated from college and married her college sweetheart. She worked in retail for five years before having the first of three children. She reports her marriage as being good overall, but strained the past few years. Despite having a successful career and high-achieving children, she reports feeling like a failure. She reports having enjoyed power walking with her friends in the past, but has stopped because of her weight gain and lack of motivation.

The family is financially stable, and her husband is a successful businessman.

Although she has social supports, she feels isolated from them. She admits to drinking more than she should over the past six months, but denies feeling out of control with her alcohol intake.

Mental status examination (MSE): Patient appears her stated age and is overweight but not obese. There is psychomotor slowing, but no abnormal motoric behavior. She is pleasant and cooperative during the interview. Her mood is depressed and affect mildly blunted. Her speech is normal. She has above average intelligence. Her cognition is good. There is no evidence of psychotic thoughts. She denies suicidal ideation or plan, but is worried how she might feel if her life does not improve. The patient's insight and judgment are intact. She feels she is depressed, but does not know how to "snap out of it." She is willing to consider any treatment recommendations except for electroconvulsive therapy (ECT).

Case discussion: This patient reports feeling much better when she is active and "making a contribution." She feels like a failure when she is not contributing to her family's well being. The patient blames herself for her children's problems and for her husband's working too hard and never being at home. She is receptive to committing to a 12-session trial of cognitive behavioral therapy (CBT) along with a specific exercise program, which she developed in consultation with her family doctor. Given her reluctance to taking medication, it was agreed that before considering taking antidepressants, she would try the therapy and exercise program for three months while closely monitoring her mental status. The patient arranged to power walk for one hour four days a week with a friend. She also joined her friend in taking tennis lessons, and joined a friendly league, with other former close friends. She was advised to *not* go on a caloric restriction diet, but rather cut out junk food, soda, high-calorie desserts and large portions. She also agreed to increase her intake of water, and limit her alcohol intake to a glass of wine with friends or with her husband at dinner, no more than 3 days per week (never drinking alone).

The patient did very well in CBT and was able to challenge her automatic belief that she was a failure. She began to understand the direct relationship between her thoughts, feelings, and behaviour. After three months she had lost six pounds, and was feeling much better about the way she felt she looked and felt. She reported starting to play tennis with her family on weekends, and planning a vacation with her husband to a major tennis tournament without her children (she reported feeling guilty about doing something for herself in the past). She was very proud of her ability to deal with her depression without having to take medication. "I'm living life again, and enjoying it," she stated at her last therapy session. She reported feeling that her success was largely due to being able to enjoy life and feel in control of her mood and behaviour. Her ability to combine her exercise with an enjoyable social interaction made adherence to her treatment program achievable and sustainable. She self-reported it made her feel more engaged in her therapy, and motivated to continue.

Why is exercise effective in treating depression?

The value of a regular physical fitness program in establishing and maintaining physical health is well established (Chakravarthy et al., 2002). The relationship between overall wellness and cardiovascular and musculoskeletal conditioning is an accepted fact and is well supported in the literature (King et al., 2009). However, the putative effect of exercise in treating major depression is less appreciated by the public and by mental health providers.

Despite major depression being a common disorder that accounts for more overall disability than any other disorder worldwide (Saveanu and Nemeroff, 2012), the precise etiology of the disorder is not known. Significant preclinical and clinical research over the past half century has yet to identify a valid and reliable diagnostic and treatment-response biomarker. Many of the core symptoms of depression overlap with other forms of psychopathology, side effects of many medications, physical illnesses, and psychosocial stressors. For example, sleep problems can be the result of physical pain, activating medications, high stress levels and anxiety, as well as a symptom of depression. Furthermore, depression is not a disorder that has a single etiologic factor; it results from a growing number of interacting biological, psychological, and social abnormalities. Emotional stress can result in a number of alterations in brain functioning, including alterations of BDNF, and neurotransmitter functioning that result in an increased risk for developing major depression. The clinical phenotype may not present until decades after the stress began, making it difficult for the patient to connect emotional stress as a cause of current symptoms.

The role of the monoamine neurotransmitters is well established as a critical causal agent, and focus of treatment intervention (Stahl and Palazidou, 1986). Virtually all of the current pharmacotherapies used to treat depression affect the presynaptic release or re-uptake of these monoamine molecules. Successful psychotherapy has recently been shown to affect brain structure and function through sophisticated neuroimaging techniques capable of demonstrating connectivity between key brain regions associated with mood (Frewen et al., 2010). Effective talk therapy is a biologic intervention, as is successful exercise therapy.

Because no single factor is the cause of major depression, it is logical that no single treatment intervention will be effective in all forms of depression. No single antibiotic treats all forms of infection. Many different treatment strategies have been shown to be effective in treating the symptoms of depression. In fact, placebo treatment can be effective in up to 30% of patients enrolled in clinical trials of antidepressant medications (Sonawalla and Rosenbaum, 2002). Exercise may have a similar placebo effect, but this does not negate the role it may play in treating depression.

Regular exercise is an important factor in maintaining good physical health. Poor health and obesity are known risk factors for depression (Craft and Landers, 1998). The reverse relationship has also been demonstrated, depression can be a risk factor for a sedentary life style (Roshanaei-Moghaddam et al., 2009). Sleep is an important factor in assessing and monitoring depression. Exercise plays a vital role in initiating maintaining restful sleep. Dyssomnia is a key factor in contributing to depressed mood, and is a risk factor, for depression (Zimmermann and Pfeiffer, 2007). Clinical research has demonstrated the role of the immune system in depression (Maes, 1999). Exercise and physical fitness play a role in maintaining optimal immune system functioning, highlighting another factor contributing to its therapeutic effect.

The psychological effects of engaging in a regular exercise program include an improved sense of self-esteem, a better sense of control over one's life, and improved focus and structure. The ability to employ a "mindfulness strategy" of focusing on the workout and staying in the moment, can be a powerful therapeutic intervention. Exercise can enhance the effects of many forms of psychotherapy proven effective in treating depression, as demonstrated in the case presented.

Finally, the positive social aspects of exercise are underappreciated. Engaging in an exercise program has the potential to create and/or strengthen a support system. Depressed patients will often isolate themselves from their support network of friends and family as a result of core symptoms of helplessness and hopelessness. As noted above, as the patient began to feel better about herself, she was able to engage in expanded social activity, like joining a tennis club. Prescribing exercise as part of treatment, not just as a leisure activity, can help motivate a depressed patient. A critical aspect of success is making sure the exercise is something the patient enjoys (or has enjoyed). The clinician needs to be creative and listen to the patient when developing a therapeutic exercise program. Ultimate success will result from a customized multimodality approach to treatment.

Case vignette: exercise as alternative to antidepressants

In a paper published in the *Harvard Health Letter* (2013), Dr. Michael Miller, discussed the impact of exercise versus antidepressants in treating depression: "For some people, [exercise] works as well as antidepressants, although exercise alone isn't enough for someone with severe depression." The following case vignette describes a patient who was able to achieve symptom relief through exercise alone.

Chief complaint / presenting symptoms: A 56-year-old man is referred for evaluation of his increasingly depressed mood, multiple somatic complaints, waking up at 3 am, low energy, lack of enjoyment in life, and isolating himself from his support network of family and friends, by his primary care physician. The patient is overweight and has elevated lipids, and is moderately hypertensive. He was reluctant to see a psychiatrist, but his primary care physician insisted he get an initial evaluation. The patient admitted to low energy, poor sleep and ongoing concern over his physical health. He reported feeling "down" much of the time, but attributed it to ongoing stress at work and in his marriage. He also disclosed a lack of libido over the past year. He denied suicidal thoughts or intent.

Past psych history: The patient denies ever being evaluated or treated by a mental health professional. He admits to periods of low mood and feeling overwhelmed in his thirties and forties, but thought "only crazy people get depression." His family doctor recommended taking an antidepressant ten years ago, but he never filled the prescription. He does not believe in psychotherapy.

Medical history: The patient has elevated blood glucose, cholesterol, and has mild hypertension. He is 20 pounds overweight and reports being a heavy snorer.

Family history: He thinks his mother suffered from depression, but was never treated, to his knowledge. His father and an uncle were heavy drinkers and may have been alcohol abusers. There was no other mental illness reported in his family.

Social history: He is a heavy social drinker, but denies drinking being a problem. He smokes 10 cigarettes a day and has cut down from a pack a day. He reports a strained relationship with his wife and very few friends at this time. He is worried about his future finances.

Mental status exam: Positive findings were depressed mood and affect blunted.

Diagnosis: The patient met diagnostic criteria for Major Depression.

Treatment recommendation and discussion: The patient did not want to start antidepressant medication and was reluctant to commit to psychotherapy. He was willing to consider starting a regular exercise program, "as this is something everybody should do." He decided to begin taking karate lessons with his adult son. After discussing his plan with his wife, she decided to join as well. Making this a family activity helped push him to attend training sessions three times a week. After six weeks of training, he had lost 12 pounds and reported an improvement in his sleep and energy levels. He felt more focused, and optimistic, in virtually all areas of his life. His libido was increasing, and his mood was elevated. As his mood gradually improved, he found it easier to discuss his life stressors and allow himself to re-engage with his family and friends. He reported that his physical health had improved, and he was able to stop many of his medications for his chronic health problems. He felt more optimistic about life over all. He agreed to return for periodic "check-ups" with his doctor to monitor his progress. This actual case highlights the importance of cognitive reframing and creating a treatment intervention a patient can accept. If his symptoms had persisted, medication and formal psychotherapy would have been necessary. In fact, the patient was engaging in nontraditional psychotherapy as a part of his karate training, which included mental training and focus exercises, along with physical conditioning. The fact that he chose karate training played an important role in the success he achieved in improving his mental and physical health.

Mechanism of action

Literature review was conducted via Google Scholar databases to ascertain the current knowledge of the role of physical exercise on mental health. The extant scientific literature proposes a number of possible mechanisms of action for exercise as a treatment for depression. Although there is no exact mechanism of action of exercise on mental health, virtually every clinical trial conducted reports significantly positive results with exercise treatment compared to control (placebo), and equal or greater effects to other treatment interventions. That said, a systematic review from 2001 cited methodological weaknesses in 17 randomized controlled trials (RCTs) from 1979 through 1999, examining exercise versus no treatment or versus established treatments for depression, highlighting the need for more research in this area (Lawlor and Hopker, 2001). However, a 2011 systematic review of 12 papers from 1985 through 2009 concluded that exercise offered a short-term improvement for patients with clinical depression and showed improved methodological quality in studies from recent years (Table 3.1) (Krogh et al., 2011).

A consistently reported mechanism has been the ability of exercise to normalize reduced levels of brain-derived neurotrophic (BDNF). This results in a neuroprotective, and possible neurotrophic effect (Seifert et al., 2010; Zschucke et al., 2013). Exercise has also been demonstrated to impact neurotransmitter functioning, especially serotonin and endorphins. Synaptic modulation of serotonin is the mechanism of action for many of the most widely prescribed antidepressants worldwide (Zschucke et al., 2013). The reports of euphoria experienced by endurance athletes, coined the runners high, has been found to result from endorphin activity directly related to mood. This is another likely mechanism of action of exercise in the treatment

Table 3.1 Summary of studies adapted from a 2011 systematic review on the effectiveness of exercise as an intervention for depression. Studies from 1997 to 2009 showed improvement in methodology. Depression scores, on average, were 0.4 of a standard deviation lower for patients completing a randomly assigned exercise intervention than for those who were not randomly assigned to receive an exercise intervention. Studies cited can be referenced from the original systematic review (Krogh et al., 2011).

Study	Type of Intervention	Percent Adherence	Results, Mean Difference (range)	Allocation Concealed	Blind	Sample Size Calc
Klein et al. (1985)	Aerobic exercise (n = 14): supervised individual running, 2×/wk; Control (n = 8): meditation in groups 1×/wk; Duration: 12 wks	55.6	SCL-D, 0.2 (−0.5 to 0.9)	No	No	No
Martinsen et al. (1985)	Aerobic exercise (n = 24): supervised group exercise 1 hr 3×/wk; Control (n = 19) occupational therapy 3×/wk; Duration: 9 wks	85.7	BDI, −10.7 (−16.3 to 5.1)	Yes	No	No
Epstein 1986	Aerobic exercise (n = 7): supervised individual running/walking 30 min 3-5x/wk; Control (n = 10): waiting list; Duration: 8 wks	Not given	BDI, −7.3 (−16.0 to 1.4)	No	No	No
Doyne et al. (1987)	Aerobic exercise (n = 8): supervised individual running/walking 4×/wk; Control (n = 11): waiting list; Duration: 8 wks	60	BDI, −7.1 (−12.3 to −1.9)	No	No	No
Mutrie (1988)	Nonaerobic exercise (n = 8): supervised individual strength training 20 min 3×/wk; Control (n = 7) waiting list; Duration: 4 wks	66	BDI, −11.9 (−16.7 to −7.1)	No	No	No
Veale et al. (1992)	Aerobic exercise (n = 36): supervised group running 3×/wk + routine care; Control (n = 29): routine care; Duration: 12 wks	75	BDI, −3.9 (−9.6 to 1.9)	Yes	No	No
Singh et al. (1997)	Nonaerobic exercise (n = 17): supervised progressive resistance training 8 reps 3 sets 3×/wk; Control (n = 15): attended health seminars; Duration: 10 wks	93	BDI, −4.0 (−10.2 to 2.2)	Yes	No	Yes
Mather et al. (2002)	Mixed aerobic and nonaerobic exercise (n = 43): supervised group exercise 45 min 3×/wk; Control (n = 43): attended health seminars; Duration: 10 wks	100	HDRS-17, −1.1 (−3.9 to 1.6)	Yes	Yes	Yes

Study	Description		Outcome			
Dunn et al. (2005)	Aerobic exercise (n = 16): individual supervised exercise 5×/wk; Control (n = 13): Flexibility exercise 3×/wk; Duration: 12 wks	72	HDRS-17, −4.0 (−7.8 to −0.2)	Yes	Yes	Yes
Singh et al. (2005)	Nonaerobic exercise (n = 18): Supervised progressive resistance training 8 reps 3 sets 3×/wk; Control (n = 19): standard treatment by general practitioner; Duration: 8 wks	90	HDRS-17, −5.9 (−9.6 to −2.2)	Yes	Yes	Yes
Blumenthal et al. (2007)	Aerobic exercise (n = 51): supervised group exercise 30 min 3×/wk; Control (n = 49): Daily placebo pills and 6 visits total by psychiatrist; Duration: 12 wks	82	HDRS-17, −1.1 (−3.6 to 1.4)	Yes	Yes	Yes
Krogh et al. (2009)	Aerobic exercise (n = 55): supervised group exercise 60 min 2×/wk; Control (n = 55): supervised group relaxation and light physical exercise for 60 min 2x/wk; Duration: 16 wks	42	HDRS-17, 0.4 (−2.0 to 2.9)	Yes	Yes	Yes

SCL-D = Symptom Check List – Depression subscale; BDI = Beck Depression Inventory; HDRS-17 = 17-item Hamilton Depression Rating Scale of depression. In addition to the biological mechanisms noted, the impact on overall psychological and social sense of well-being likely contribute to its putative effects as well (Read and Brown, 2003; Stathopoulou et al., 2006). Given the clinical reports of effectiveness and the clinical research findings, exercise should be considered as a potential treatment modality for depression in patients of all ages, particularly given its low-side-effect profile compared to other treatments for depression.

Side-effect profile

One of the most desirable aspects of employing exercise as a treatment intervention in depression is its very low-side-effect profile compared to pharmacologic treatments. In fact, exercise is one of the only treatments that actually improves overall physical health and self-reported health-related quality of life (Schmitz et al., 2004).

The potential side effects of existing treatment options for depression are extensive and well documented. Antidepressant medications have been the mainstay of treatment for depression for the past 35 years. Antidepressants are effective in treating depression in over 60% of treated patients, but are often hampered by their side-effect profiles (Peretti et al., 2000). The original tricyclic antidepressants (TCAs) were (and are) effective medications in treating depression, but their side-effect profile often resulted in patients prematurely discontinuing the medication. Commonly occurring side effects, such as dry mouth, constipation, and significant weight gain, resulted in discontinuation by the patient before the drug had a chance to be effective. Antidepressant medications require a minimum of three to five weeks of daily use, at the therapeutic dose, before clinical improvement is experienced. Later-generation antidepressants were able to eliminate the weight gain and dry mouth, but had their own adverse side effects. These included upset stomach and loss of libido, again contributing to early termination of taking the medication and a return of depressive symptoms. A meta-analysis comparing the side effects of tricyclic antidepressants (TCAs) with serotonin reuptake inhibitors (SSRIs), demonstrated clinically significant adverse effects, with 27% of patients experiencing dry mouth from TCA use and 26% experiencing nausea from SSRI use.

Potential side effects of exercise treatment include a risk of developing sport-related musculoskeletal injury and the small risk of developing exercise addiction (Lauer, 2006). Exercise addiction occurs rarely, presenting in 3% of the general population (Sussman et al., 2011) Exercise addiction is hallmarked by a patient continuing to over-exercise, even when faced with physical injury and/or personal inconvenience and disruption in daily life. Like other forms of addictive behaviors, the obsessive aspect of overengaging/overusing is not a common component of depression, but rather an obsessive disorder. Exercise addiction should be conceptualized and treated like other obsessive disorders.

This is not a primary mood disorder, although it could be a co-morbid condition.

Optimal treatment for depression is often best achieved with a combination of treatment interventions. Extant literature clearly documents the important additive effect of medication and psychotherapy for moderate to severe depression. Given its benefit in maintaining mental and physical health, well supervised exercise should be recommended to all depressed patients. The benefits of adding an enjoyable exercise program to all treatment strategies is highly recommended for all patients suffering from depression. A final clinical case vignette will address this aspect of exercise therapy.

Case vignette: exercise alongside CBT alleviates depression, weight gain, and hypertension

The following case highlights the value of combined treatment modalities when treating depression.

A 38-year-old man is referred to a psychiatrist for a consultation requesting a second opinion on treatment of depression. The patient has been diagnosed with major depression for the past three years. For the past two and a half years he has been taking an antidepressant prescribed by his primary care physician. The patient reports he has been able to return to work, but is not able to function at the same level he was before becoming depressed. He continues to struggle with the fear his depression will return. He reports a positive family history for depression in his father and an uncle. His father never sought formal treatment, and self-medicated with alcohol for many years.

Although he was advised to seek psychotherapy by his primary care physician, the patient has resisted. He sees no value in "sharing his dirty laundry" with someone else, and does not want to spend the money or time seeing a therapist. He has also refused going to a psychiatrist, but is willing to get an opinion on possible medication changes. His initial history confirms the diagnosis of major depression recurrent, in partial remission.

The suggestion to reconsider psychotherapy was presented during the consult. The patient reported he was not interested in discussing "how I feel about my mother," or "discussing his sexual interests." This was his belief of what psychotherapy would entail. When informed that therapy comes in many different forms, many focusing on current issues in his life and how to better handle stress, he was willing to reconsider his decision.

The important role of exercise as part of his treatment was also discussed. The patient expressed concern over his health, as he reported significant weight gain since starting antidepressant medication. He believes the weight gain was related to his lack of exercise and poor eating habits. The patient felt that getting regular exercise was a luxury he could not afford. Hearing that this was a critical component of his treatment, and not a luxury, allowed him to reframe his thoughts on making exercise a treatment for both his physical and mental health.

Six months after the consult, the psychiatrist contacted the referring primary care physician to get follow up on the patient condition. The primary care physician reported the patient had lost 20 pounds and was no longer on medication for mild hypertension. He had completed a 12-week CBT therapy program, and was a regular at the gym where he had made new friends.

The patient's concept of psychotherapy needed to be clarified. He also needed the doctors to give him permission to include exercise as part of his treatment, reframing it from being a recreational activity. The addition of an exercise program to his treatment plan provided an additive therapeutic effect for his mood and his physical health. The ability to cut down on medications that may have been contributing to his lack of energy was also a positive effect of adding exercise to his treatment. Exercise permitted the patient to take a more active role in his treatment, adding to his recovering self-confidence and sense of control of his life stressors.

Conclusion

The goal of this chapter was to educate the reader about the role of exercise in treating depression. Current American Psychiatric Association practice guidelines include exercise as an important adjunct in the treatment of depression. Clinical research has demonstrated the effectiveness of exercise as a treatment modality, and offers a mechanism of action for its therapeutic effectiveness. Clinical investigators at University of Texas Southwestern, who conducted the Treatment with Exercises Augmentation for Depression (TREAD) study, concluded that exercise is "important in treating depression" (Trivedi et al., 2006). This National Institute of Mental Health–funded research played a pivotal role in the APA practice guideline recommendations. It demonstrated that aerobic exercise, at high and low "doses," resulted in reduced levels of the pro-inflammatory cytokines interleukin-1B (IL-1beta) and tumor necrosis factor-alpha (TNF-alpha). Both of these are elevated in patients with major depression, making them potential biomarkers for depression treatment response.

Is exercise effective in curing every patient with depression? The answer is no, but no single treatment intervention has been demonstrated to achieve this result. The growing body of clinical research supports the role of exercise as an effective therapeutic intervention, both as a primary and adjunctive therapy. When properly supervised, there are few treatment options that offer a safer side-effect profile, and added physical and emotional health benefits. In fact, few, if any, treatments offer the overall health promotion of physical exercise. Additional research is needed to better determine how to achieve the maximal therapeutic effect of exercise treatment for depressed patients of all ages and both genders. The type of exercise, aerobic vs. resistance training, the amount and timing of the exercise, and other clinical variables, are all questions that need to be researched in well controlled, well designed future clinical trials.

References

Chakravarthy MV, Joyner MJ and Booth FW (2002) An obligation for primary care physicians to prescribe physical activity to sedentary patients to reduce the risk of chronic health conditions. *Mayo Clinic Proceedings* 77(2): 165–173.

Craft LL and Landers DM (1998) The effect of exercise on clinical depression and depression resulting from mental illness: a meta analysis. *Journal of Sport and Exercise Psychology* 20: 339–357.

Duncan TE and McAuley E (1993) Social support and efficacy cognitions in exercise adherence: a latent growth curve analysis. *Journal of Behavioral Medicine* 16(2): 199–218.

Exercise is an all-natural treatment to fight depression (2013) Harvard Health Letter. Aug 2013: 3

Frewen PA, Dozois DJ and Lanius RA (2010) Neuroimaging studies of psychological interventions for mood and anxiety disorders: empirical and methodological review. *FOCUS: The Journal of Lifelong Learning in Psychiatry* 8(1): 92–109.

Grant M (1991) *A Short History of Classical Civilization*. London: Weidenfeld and Nicolson.

King NA, Hopkins M, Caudwell P, et al. (2009) Beneficial effects of exercise: shifting the focus from body weight to other markers of health. *British Journal of Sports Medicine* 43(12): 924–927.

Krogh J, Nordentoft M, Sterne JA et al. (2011) The effect of exercise in clinically depressed adults: systematic review and meta-analysis of randomized controlled trials. *Journal of Clinical Psychiatry* 72(4): 529–538.

Lauer H (2006) *The new Americans: defining ourselves through sports and fitness participation*. Boston, MA: American Sports Data Inc.

Lawlor DA and Hopker SW (2001) The effectiveness of exercise as an intervention in the management of depression: systematic review and meta-regression analysis of randomized controlled trials. *British Medical Journal* 322: 1–8.

Maes M (1999) Major depression and activation of the inflammatory response system. *Advances in Experimental Medicine* 461: 25–46.

Marcus MM, Yaghi MY, van Ommeren M et al. (2012) WHO Department of Mental Health and Substance Abuse. *Depression: A Global Public Health Concern*. Available at: http://www.who.int/entity/mental_health/manage ment/depression/who_paper_depression_wfmh_2012.pdf?ua=1.

National Collaborating Centre for Mental Health (2010) *Depression: the NICE guideline on the treatment and management of depression in adults (Updated edition)*. London: RCPsych Publications.

Peretti S, Judge R and Hindmarch I (2000) Safety and tolerability considerations: tricyclic antidepressants vs. selective serotonin reuptake inhibitors. *Acta Psychiatrica Scandinavica* 101(S403): 17–25.

Read J and Brown R (2003) The Role of Physical Exercise in Alcoholism. *Prof Psychol Res Pract* 34(1):49–56.

Roshanaei-Moghaddam B, Katon WJ and Russo J (2009) The longitudinal effects of depression on physical activity. *General Hospital Psychiatry* 31(4): 306–315.

Saveanu RV and Nemeroff CB (2012) Etiology of depression: genetic and environmental factors. *Psychiatric Clinics of North America* 35(1): 51–71.

Sonawalla SB and Rosenbaum JF (2002) Placebo response in depression. *Dialogues in Clinical Neuroscience* 4(1): 105–113.

Stahl SM and Palazidou L (1986) The pharmacology of depression: studies of neurotransmitter receptors lead the search for biochemical lesions and new drug therapies. *Trends in Pharmacological Sciences* 7: 349–354.

Stathopoulou G, Powers M et al. (2006) Exercise interventions for mental health: a quantitative and qualitative review *Clin Psychol Sci Pract* 13(2):179–193.

Sussman S, Lisha N and Griffiths M (2011) Prevalence of the addictions: a problem of the majority or the minority? *Evaluation & the Health Professions* 34: 3–56.

Trivedi MH, Greer TL, Grannemann BD et al. (2006) TREAD: TReatment with Exercise Augmentation for Depression: study rationale and design. *Clinical Trials* 3(3): 291–305.

Waraich P, Goldner EM, Somers JM et al. (2004) Prevalence and incidence studies of mood disorders: a systematic review of the literature. *Canadian Journal of Psychiatry* 49: 124–138.

Zimmermann C and Pfeiffer H (2007) Sleep disorders in depression: suggestions for a therapeutic approach. *Der Nervenarzt* 78(1): 21–30.

Zschucke E, Gaudlitz K, Strohle A (2013) Exercise and Physical Activity in Mental Disorders: Clinical and Experimental Evidence. *J Prev Med Public Health* 46: s12–21.

4

Activity intervention for first-episode psychosis

Eric Y. H. Chen, Jingxia Lin and Edwin H. M. Lee

Summary

Physical inactivity is a major contributor to death and disability from non-communicable diseases, including diseases of the heart and vascular system, diabetes mellitus, cancers, and obstructive pulmonary disease. Physical inactivity is also associated with poorer cognitive functioning, increased risks of global cognitive decline, and quality of life in various mental illnesses. People with first-episode psychosis present a challenging group for early intervention, as optimal treatment would have long-term impact on functioning and outcomes. Significant cognitive benefits from regular aerobic exercise and mind-body exercise are noted in attention, processing speed, executive function, and working memory. Physical exercise is a non-invasive non-pharmacological intervention which is good for physical, psychological and social aspects. It reduces the potential risks of cardiovascular and metabolic diseases, and improves cognition and physiological functions of the brain. The chapter will offer first-hand experience about exercise intervention in people with first-episode psychosis, and will share clinical experiences in exercise research and promotion of exercise.

Key points

Physical inactivity is related to cognitive deficits, increased risks of metabolic disorders and poor quality of life in first-episode psychosis patients.

Physical exercise enhances cognitive functions (e.g., memory and attention) and improves clinical outcomes in patients with psychosis.

Physical Exercise Interventions for Mental Health, ed. Linda C. W. Lam and Michelle Riba. Published by Cambridge University Press. © Cambridge University Press 2016.

Physical exercise should be promoted in clinical practice as a non-invasive adjunctive treatment which is good for physical, psychological and social functioning.

Tips and advice for patients

Know yourself before exercising: Examine health conditions before starting to do exercise. Pay attention to the contraindications to vigorous physical exercise, such as myocardial infarction, hypertension, and spinal and joint problems, and arrange suitable exercise for yourself.

Do it in short bouts: Moderate-intensity physical exercise can be accumulated throughout the day in 10-minute bouts, which is as effective as exercising for 30 minutes straight. This is useful when trying to fit exercise into a busy schedule.

Mix it up: Combinations of different types of exercise can be used to make more fun. For example, you can do aerobic exercise for 15 minutes and yoga for 15 minutes afterwards; or you can run for 30 minutes twice per week and play basketball on two other days.

Set your schedule: The recommended exercise frequency is 30 minutes per session, and three sessions per week. It is important to set aside specific days and times for exercise, making it just as much a regular part of your schedule as eating and sleeping.

Do exercise everywhere: The gymnasium is not a necessity. A pair of athletic shoes and a little motivation are all you need to live a more active and healthier life.

Make it a family affair: Take your partner, your children or your friends with you during exercise to add some fun and motivation to your routine.

Physical inactivity causes 6–10% of the non-communicable diseases including cardiovascular disease, diabetes, and breast and colon cancer (Lee et al., 2012). Furthermore, this unhealthy behavior is associated with cognitive deficits, impaired functioning and poor quality of life in patients with mental health issues (Buchman et al., 2012; D. Vancampfort et al., 2013). A recent study examined the association between physical activity levels and functioning in patients with first-episode psychosis, and found that patients who were physically inactive had more positive and negative symptoms (Lee et al., 2013). Weuve and colleagues (2004) examined the relation of regular physical exercise to cognitive function and found that higher levels of activity were associated with better cognitive performance. Another study suggested that high levels of physical activity were associated with reduced risks of cognitive impairment, Alzheimer disease and dementia of any type (Laurin, Verreault, Lindsay, MacPherson, & Rockwood, 2001).

People with schizophrenia and related disorders are more likely to be physically inactive than healthy populations as a consequence of the disorder (Lindamer et al., 2008), and metabolic syndrome and cardiovascular risk factors are highly prevalent in this population (De Hert et al., 2011). It has been recognized that obesity is 1.5 to 2 times more prevalent in schizophrenic patients than in the general population, and the risk for diabetes and hypertension is 2 times higher than in normal people (De Hert, Schreurs, Vancampfort, & Van Winkel, 2009). People with first-episode psychosis present a challenging group for early intervention, as antipsychotic treatment induces weight gain and metabolic inference which have long-term impact on functioning and disease outcomes (Graham et al., 2005; Strassnig, Miewald, Keshavan & Ganguli, 2007).

Clinical impacts of physical exercise for psychosis

A systematic review on exercise and patients with schizophrenia and related disorders by Vancampfort and colleagues (2009) concluded that physical exercise was feasible and efficacious in reducing weight and decreasing the risk of obesity-related cardiovascular diseases. Beebe and colleagues(2005) reported increased aerobic fitness and decreased body mass index in the experimental group over the exercise period compared with the control group. Similar findings regarding improvement of aerobic fitness and muscular fitness were also reported by Marzolini and colleagues (2009). In contrast, the enhancement of the maximal oxygen uptake after a 12-week cycling programme in chronic schizophrenic patients was not significant compared with the control conditions (Pajonk et al., 2010).

Benefits of physical exercise in clinical symptoms have been robustly reported during recent years. A few systematic reviews demonstrated that both aerobic exercise (Ellis, Crone, Davey, & Grogan, 2007; Faulkner & Biddle, 1999; Holley, Crone, Tyson, & Lovell, 2011; Vancampfort, Knapen, et al., 2012) and mind-body exercise (Balasubramaniam, Telles, & Doraiswamy, 2012; Vancampfort, Vansteelandt, et al., 2012) significantly reduced clinical signs and attenuated secondary symptoms in patients with schizophrenia and psychosis, such as depression, self-depreciation and social withdrawal. Two robust studies examining the effectiveness of aerobic exercise in schizophrenic patients found a significant reduction in the psychiatric symptoms after a 16-week training programme (Beebe et al., 2005; Duraiswamy, Thirthalli, Nagendra, & Gangadhar, 2007) (Table 4.1).

Besides aerobic exercise, yoga therapy has been increasingly used to ameliorate the symptoms and emotional deficits in schizophrenia. Two review papers of three randomized controlled clinical trials (RCTs) with high methodological quality examined the effects of yoga on schizophrenia (Balasubramaniam et al., 2012; Vancampfort, Vansteelandt, et al., 2012). Significant reductions in the Positive and Negative Syndrome Scale (PANSS) total score, positive syndrome, negative syndrome and general psychopathology subscores were observed in subjects with schizophrenia spectrum disorders treated with yoga compared with wait-list controls (Behere et al., 2011; Visceglia & Lewis, 2011) or with the stretching exercise group (Duraiswamy et al., 2007). The intervention period varied from 8 weeks to 16 weeks, and the duration of training with an instructor varied from 3 weeks to 8 weeks. A recent RCT compared the therapeutic efficacy

Table 4.1 *Overview Details of Aerobic Exercise clinical trials in Schizophrenia*

Study	Subjects	Interventions	Duration	Frequency	Control Condition	Relevant Outcomes
Beebe et al. (2005)	10 outpatients with schizophrenia; aged 40–63y	Aerobic exercise (treadmill walking)	16 weeks	From 25 min 3 times/wk (wk1) to 50 min 3 times/wk (wk3 to end)	Care as usual	Fewer positive and negative symptoms (−13.5% vs. +5%, p<.05)
Beebe et al. (2013)	22 outpatients with schizophrenia or schizoaffective disorder; aged 23–71 y (mean age = 48.1y)	Follow-up patients after exercise intervention (Walking with pedometers)	14–34 mo (mean 22 mo)	Daily steps ranged from 64 to 13463 (mean = 4425 steps)	Follow-up patients in non-exercise group	Experimental subjects walked more steps and covered more distance than controls
Behere et al. (2011)	66 outpatients with schizophrenia; mean age = 31.8y	Aerobic and muscle strength exercises vs yoga	3 mo	60-min sessions in wk 1–4 under supervision and then 3 mo of self-practice	Waiting list	Significant fewer positive and negative symptom scores (p<.01) only 2 and 4 mo after yoga, respectively; reductions after aerobic and muscle strength not significant
Chen et al. (2009)	18 inpatients with schizophrenia; mean age = 40y	PMR	11 d	40 min/d	Care as usual	Less anxiety after 11d (p<.001) and 1 wk later (−65%, p<.045 vs −13% in controls)
Duraiswamy et al. (2007)	41 inpatients and outpatients with schizophrenia; aged 18–55y	Aerobic and strength exercises	16 wk	60 min 5 times/wk in wk 1–3 under supervision and then 3 mo of self-practice	yoga	Fewer positive and negative symptoms after aerobic and strength exercises (group difference p = .24 and p<.01)
Hawkins et al. (1980)	40 inpatients with schizophrenia; mean age = 35y	PMR vs thermal feedback vs PMR+thermal feedback	2 wk	40 min 5 times/wk	Minimal treatment	Reductions across groups for state anxiety (p<.05); reductions associated with fewer hospitalization at 1-y follow-up (p<.05)

Study	Participants	Intervention	Duration	Session frequency	Control	Results
Marzolini et al. (2009)	13 inpatients and outpatients with schizophrenia or schizoaffective disorder; mean age = 44.6y	Aerobic and muscle strength exercises	12 wk	90 min 2 times/wk	Care as usual	6MWT score +5.1% (vs −5.5% in controls); muscle strength +28.3% (vs +12.5% in controls, $p<.001$); no significant reductions in resting blood pressure or BMI
Pajonk et al. (2010)	16 male outpatients with schizophrenia; aged 20–51y	Aerobic exercises (cycling)	3 mo	30 min 3 times/wk	Table football	STM improved by 34% ($p<.01$); HV and VO2max/kg increased after exercise ($p<.002$ and $p = .35$); STM and VO2max correlated with HV ($r = .51$, $p<.05$ and $r = .71$, $p<.01$)
Pharr & Coursey (1989)	30 inpatients with schizophrenia; mean age = 35y	PMR vs EMG biofeedback	20 min	7 individual sessions	Listening to recorded readings	No significant changes in tension-anxiety scores
Vancampfort et al. (2011)	40 inpatients with schizophrenia or schizoaffective disorder; mean age = 32.77y	Aerobic exercise vs yoga	30 min of yoga and 20 min of cycling	Single session	Resting control condition	Reduced state anxiety ($p<.001$) and psychological distress ($p<.001$) after yoga and aerobic exercise but not after control condition
Vancampfort et al. (2011)	52 inpatients with schizophrenia; mean age = 35.6y	PMR	25 min	Single session	Reading control condition	Reduced state anxiety ($p<.001$) and psychological distress ($p<.001$) after PMR but not after control condition

PMR = progressive muscle relaxation; BMI = body mass index; 6MWT = Six-Minute Walk Test; STM = short-term memory; HV = hippocampal volume; VO2max = maximum oxygen consumption.

of yoga with exercise and wait-list controls in stabilized schizophrenic outpatients. Similar improvements in PANSS total and negative subscore as well as social functioning score were reported in yoga therapy group (Varambally et al., 2012).

Vancampfort and colleagues (2011) found that a single session of aerobic exercise can significantly reduce anxiety state, psychological distress, and improve subjective well-being in schizophrenic patients. Similarly, a single 30-minute yoga session in patients with schizophrenia or related disorders resulted in significantly decreased state anxiety and psychological stress, and increased subjective well-being with large effect sizes compared to the control (Vancampfort, De Hert, Knapen, Wampers, et al., 2011). In addition, several studies have examined the effectiveness of a progressive muscle relaxation programme for schizophrenic patients. Significant reductions in anxiety state and psychological distress were observed, which correlated with fewer hospitalizations (Hawkins, Doell, Lindseth, Jeffers, & Skaggs, 1980; Vancampfort, De Hert, Knapen, Maurissen, et al., 2011).

The benefit of physical exercise in neurocognition has been rarely explored in psychotic disorders. Cognitive dysfunction is a core feature of psychosis, but pharmacological treatments have limited effects. Recently, an RCT investigated chronic schizophrenic patients on a 12-week cycling programme to assess the cognitive impacts of aerobic exercise. A significant improvement in the test scores for short-term memory was observed, which was associated with the increase in hippocampal volume (Pajonk et al., 2010). Patients practicing yoga for 12 or 16 weeks demonstrated significant improvement in facial emotion recognition impairments and socio-occupational functioning (Behere et al., 2011; Duraiswamy et al., 2007). A recent study in Hong Kong investigated the effects of aerobic exercise and yoga on neurocognition and clinical symptoms for patients with early psychosis. After practicing three sessions for 12 weeks, both types of exercise improved short-term and long-term memory, as well as working memory. Yoga has been found to be effective in improving attention and concentration. Moreover, both types of exercise eliminated positive and negative symptoms, as well as depressive symptoms compared to a wait-list control group.

No adverse events due to physical exercise were reported in any of these studies, although the procedure for reporting adverse events was variable across the studies. All the published studies mentioned above indicated that physical exercise is a non-invasive non-pharmacological intervention which is good for physical, psychological and social aspects.

Potential mechanisms for the benefits of physical exercise

Neurogenesis
Neurogenesis is the generation of new neurons and usually occurs in the olfactory bulb and dentate gyrus of the hippocampus in the adult mammalian brain (van Praag, 2009). This process has been proven to be highly associated with learning and memory, and is regulated by many extrinsic and intrinsic environmental factors (Taupin, 2006). Large numbers of animal studies suggest that physical

exercise strongly stimulates neurogenesis in the hippocampus, resulting in an improvement of hippocampus-related cognitive functions (van Praag, Christie, Sejnowski, & Gage, 1999; van Praag, Kempermann, & Gage, 1999). Research on wheel-running rats indicates a positive correlation between running and neurogenesis in the dentate gyrus of the hippocampus, which was associated with learning ability (van Praag, 2008). Conversely, recent animal studies have proposed that neurogenesis inhibition improved learning and memory performance (Kerr, Steuer, Pochtarev, & Swain, 2010), or that neurogenesis was selectively associated with improvement in cognitive performances (Clark et al., 2008). Although promoting hippocampal neurogenesis by physical exercise is a highly reproducible effect, the mechanism of how hippocampal neurogenesis supports behavioural improvements is still controversial.

Additionally, the structural changes following exercise were also reflected in the enhancement of synaptic plasticity and properties of dendritic spines (van Praag, 2009). Both voluntary and forced exercise enhanced the expression of long-term potentiation (LTP) specifically in the dentate gyrus of the hippocampus, and enhanced object recognition learning ability in rodents (Farmer et al., 2004; O'Callaghan, Ohle, & Kelly, 2007). LTP induction is associated with changes in dendritic spine size and quantity, which are speculated to support synaptic strength changes (van Praag, 2009). An in vivo rat study showed long-term voluntary running significantly increased the dendritic spine density in the entorhinal cortex layer III, area CA1 and dentate gyrus of the hippocampus (Redila & Christie, 2006; Stranahan, Khalil, & Gould, 2007). Physical activity was also found to accelerate the maturation of dendritic spines in newborn neurons (Zhao, Teng, Summers, Ming, & Gage, 2006).

Angiogenesis and vascular changes

Spirduso (1980) speculated that regular physical exercise changed cognition by increasing cerebral blood flow (CBF). Recent promising developments in the study of cerebral metabolic responses to physical activity have also uncovered information regarding the blood flow in specific vessels, blood flow velocity, cerebral tissue oxygenation and metabolism (Gonzalez-Alonso et al., 2004; Ide, Horn, & Secher, 1999; Lojovich, 2010). Regional CBF is increased by up to 30% from rest to the maximal aerobic exercise level as indicated in both animal and human studies. The enhanced CBF was observed in the middle and anterior cerebral arteries (Christensen et al., 2000; Jorgensen, Perko, Hanel, Schroeder, & Secher, 1992).

Angiogenesis, the growth of new blood vessels, is also linked to enhanced learning and memory (Creer, Romberg, Saksida, van Praag, & Bussey, 2010; Kerr et al., 2010; Pereira et al., 2007). Black and colleagues(1990) were the first to show long-term physical exercise could achieve a longer lasting effect on CBF by increasing capillary density and perfusion in the primary motor cortex of rodents. Unlike neurogenesis, angiogenesis induced by aerobic exercise occurred just outside of the hippocampus, and were distributed in the cerebellum (Black et al., 1990; Isaacs, Anderson, Alcantara, Black, & Greenough, 1992) and primary motor cortex (Kleim, Cooper, & VandenBerg, 2002; Swain et al., 2003). Furthermore, findings from two animal studies suggest that exercise-related increases in hippocampal angiogenesis only occurred in young rats but not old rats (Creer et al., 2010; van Praag, Shubert, Zhao, & Gage, 2005). For example, a study by Creer and colleagues (2010) showed moderate improvement in performance without significant hippocampal angiogenesis in aged rats aerobically trained. A human study by Timinkul (2008) also revealed that mild physical exercise had an enhancing effect on cerebral blood flow in healthy young men. The role of angiogenesis related to aerobic training in cognitive functions across a life span is still a topic that needs further research.

Structural brain changes induced by exercise

In vivo animal and human studies indicate that exercise improves hippocampus-dependent learning and memory by enhancing hippocampal neurogenesis (Clark et al., 2008; Shors et al., 2001; 2002; van Praag, 2008). Increasing evidence shows that physical exercise can increase brain volume, particularly in the hippocampus where impressive increases have been demonstrated. A recent research study observed a significant increase in hippocampal volume in both patients with chronic schizophrenia and healthy controls following a 12-week cycling programme. The hippocampal increase was significantly correlated with an improvement in short-term memory (Pajonk et al., 2010). Using MRI-based cortical pattern matching to investigate grey matter density and brain surface expansion in healthy controls revealed significantly increased grey matter density in the right frontal and occipital pole regions (Falkai et al., 2012). Erickson and colleagues (2011) found that the hippocampal volume increased by 2% in elderly subjects following a 1 to 2-year exercise programme. Exercise selectively increased the volume of the hippocampus, which was accompanied by an increase in serum brain-derived neurotrophic factor (BDNF) levels. BDNF is a member of the neurotrophin family; its significance in neurogenesis will be reviewed below. Studies in pre-adolescent children have shown that increases in bilateral hippocampal volume mediated by fitness level were also linked to relational memory (Chaddock et al., 2010). Studies in both animals and humans have indicated that aerobic exercise selectively increased the anterior hippocampus volume, which contains the dentate gyrus subregion associated with neurogenesis, but no volumetric changes were observed in the posterior hippocampus, thalamus or caudate nucleus (Erickson et al., 2011; Farmer et al., 2004; Pereira et al., 2007).

In addition to the hippocampus, some studies showed significant changes in other brain regions following aerobic exercise. Research in rodents suggests that wheel running can change the molecular architecture and function of the basal ganglia. The basal ganglia, a group of structures at the base of the forebrain subdivided into the dorsal and ventral striatum, are involved in motor control, cognitive flexibility, learning and affective functions (Aron, Poldrack, & Wise, 2009; Casey, Getz, & Galvan, 2008; Graybiel, 2005). A cross-sectional study in pre-adolescent children indicated that improved cognitive control induced by aerobic fitness was associated with an increase in the dorsal striatum (Chaddock et al., 2010). A study by Colcombe and colleagues (2006) on healthy senile subjects following an aerobic programme for 6 months, demonstrated increases in grey matter volume in the inferior frontal gyrus, anterior cingulate and superior temporal gyrus, and an increase in anterior white matter volume. In another RCT of older adults who were taught to juggle, significant increases in the grey matter in the middle temporal area of the visual cortex, and transient increases in the grey matter in hippocampus and nucleus accumbens were observed in the juggling group compared with control group (Boyke, Driemeyer, Gaser, Buchel, & May, 2008). The study conducted in early psychotic patients in Hong Kong indicated that cortical thickness of the superior frontal gyrus increased after 12-week aerobic exercise, and cortical thickness of post-central gyrus increased after 12-week yoga intervention.

The majority of imaging studies looking at the brain changes induced by yoga focused on the effects of meditation combined with controlled breathing. Meditation is one of the main components of yoga, which is usually achieved with focused breathing and clearing of the mind. The neurological mechanisms underlying meditation have been widely explored using advanced imaging techniques. Changes to cerebral blood flow during Iyengar yoga training, which involves body movements and meditation, were examined in experienced practitioners using single-photon emission computed tomography (SPECT). Significant decreases of the pre- and post-intervention CBF ratio were observed in the right amygdala, right dorsal medial cortex and right sensorimotor areas. Significant increases of the pre- and post-intervention CBF ratio were observed in the bilateral dorsal medial frontal lobe, right prefrontal cortex, right sensorimotor cortex, right inferior and superior frontal lobes (Cohen et al., 2009).

Increasing numbers of imaging studies have examined the morphological differences between meditation practitioners and controls from the normal population. The study by Lazar and colleagues compared the cortical thickness of Buddhist insight meditation practitioners with matched controls. They found significantly thicker cortices in the right anterior insula and the right middle and superior frontal sulci of the meditators (Lazar et al., 2005). Pagnoni and Cekic observed a trend of increasing grey matter volume in the left putamen in Zen meditation practitioners, and this neuroprotective effect correlated with less impairment in target sensitivity and speed of responses (Pagnoni & Cekic, 2007). Similar to the findings of Lazar and colleagues, the study by Holzel and colleagues reported increases in the grey matter concentration in the right anterior insula of advanced meditators. In addition, they found significantly higher concentrations of grey matter in the left inferior temporal gyrus and right hippocampus (Holzel et al., 2008). Results consistent with Holzel and colleagues were reported by Luders and colleagues, who compared 22 long-term practitioners of different types of meditation with 22 matched controls. The meditators had increased grey matter in the left inferior temporal gyrus, right hippocampus, right orbito-frontal gyrus and in the right thalamus (Luders, Toga, Lepore, & Gaser, 2009). Finally, another Danish study focusing on Tibetan meditation, which focuses on breathing and teaches an open and positive attitude, found a higher concentration of grey matter in the prefrontal cortex and anterior lobe of the cerebellum, as well as in the medulla oblongata (Vestergaard-Poulsen et al., 2009).

Functional Brain Changes Induced by Exercise

The effects of physical exercise on brain activity during a cognitive task or resting state provide some interesting insights into brain functions. Studies using event-related potentials (ERPs) have suggested that higher aerobic fitness levels are associated with larger P300s during information processing in preadolescent subjects (Hillman, Castelli, & Buck, 2005; Pontifex et al., 2011). P300 is an ERP component that is thought to emerge from the temporoparietal cortex, and whose amplitude is related to attention and concentration (Polich, 2007). Using the Eriksen flanker task, both children and young adults with high fitness levels showed a smaller error-related negativity (ERN), an ERP component that indexes conflict monitoring and error evaluation, and larger error positivity (Pe), an ERP component that indexes awareness of one's own mistakes (Hillman et al., 2009; Themanson & Hillman, 2006).

With the development of the functional magnetic resonance imaging (fMRI) techniques, more robust evidence of the activity and connectivity of the brain has been published. In a cross-sectional study, differences in brain activity during processing of congruent and incongruent cognitive tasks were found to be associated with cardiorespiratory fitness levels of the subjects. Subjects with greater fitness levels demonstrated increased activity in the right dorsolateral prefrontal cortex and relatively reduced activity in the anterior cingulate cortex during a flanker task, in which the subjects were asked to respond to a central arrow cue embedded in a series of five arrows pointing either to the left or right (Colcombe et al., 2004). This result suggested that aerobic exercise may lead to improved top-down control from the prefrontal cortex involved in conflict regulation performance (Botvinick, Braver, Barch, Carter, & Cohen, 2001). Connectivity in the brain refers to how different brain areas communicate with each other under certain cognitive demands or in the resting state. Voss and colleagues(2010) examined whether long-term regular aerobic exercise would enhance the connectivity in the Default Network, which is a network involving several brain regions proven to be associated with attention and self-awareness, or enhance connectivity in other brain networks responsible for higher-level executive functions, spatial attention, motor control and audition. Improved connectivity was observed primarily in the Default Network of senile participants after a one-year aerobic training programme, further connectivity increases were found between bilateral prefrontal cortices in an Executive Control network. This robust evidence suggests that both brain activation and connectivity of brain networks benefit from aerobic exercise.

Functional brain mapping during meditation has also been increasingly explored. An early trial investigated the brain activity during a single meditation session in a small sample of healthy subjects. Significantly increased signals were observed in several brain regions involved in attention and memory functions, namely the dorsolateral prefrontal and parietal cortices, hippocampus/parahippocampus, temporal lobe, anterior cingulate cortex, striatum, and pre- and post-central gyri. Moreover, globally decreased fMRI signals were observed in one subject, which was probably secondary to cardiorespiratory alteration (Lazar et al., 2000). Engstrom and colleagues conducted a cross-sectional fMRI study during silent mantra meditation in eight subjects who had practiced meditation for less than two years. The most significant activated signals were observed in the bilateral hippocampal/parahippocampal formations, and increased activation was also observed in other regions including bilateral middle cingulate cortex and bilateral precentral cortex (Engstrom, Pihlsgard, Lundberg, & Soderfeldt, 2010). Furthermore, Engstrom and colleagues did not find any activation in the anterior cingulate cortex, and only a small activation was observed in the prefrontal cortex, which was contrary to the study by Lazar and colleagues. Recent neural network research has suggested that the limbic/paralimbic-bulbar circuitry, including the anterior cingulate, amygdala and anterior insular cortices, plays a vital role in cognitive and emotional modulation of spontaneous breathing (Evans et al., 2009). Kilpatrick and colleagues conducted an RCT in healthy female subjects who were trained in a mindfulness-based stress reduction programme (MBSR) for eight weeks, and reported significant MBSR-related differences in functional connectivity, mainly in the auditory/salience and medial visual networks (Kilpatrick et al., 2011). The authors concluded that the eight-week mindfulness-based meditation changed intrinsic functional connectivity that resulted in more consistent concentration, improved sensory processing, and reflective awareness of sensory experience (Kilpatrick et al., 2011).

Brain-derived neurotrophic factor (BDNF)

Robust research findings have suggested that several candidates from circulating neurochemicals may mediate the cognitive benefits associated with physical exercise in both animal and human beings. BDNF and IGF-1 are two candidates that are most promising from recent empirical studies. BDNF is a member of the neurotrophin family, which is known to play a prominent role in the differentiation, extension, survival, growth and maintenance of neurons throughout the brain. This basic protein is present at high concentrations in the hippocampus, which is an area associated with learning and memory ability (Barde, 1994; Leibrock et al., 1989). BDNF modulates synaptic plasticity by regulating branching and remodelling in axons and dendrites (Lom & Cohen-Cory, 1999), synaptogenesis in axon arborization (Alsina, Vu, & Cohen-Cory, 2001), synaptic transmission efficacy (Lohof, Ip, & Poo, 1993), and the excitatory and inhibitory synaptogenesis (Rutherford, Nelson, & Turrigiano, 1998; Seil & Drake-Baumann, 2000). A single intense bout of exercise (Ferris, Williams, & Shen, 2007; Rasmussen et al., 2009) or long-term regular aerobic exercise (Neeper, Gomez-Pinilla, Choi, & Cotman, 1996; Zoladz et al., 2008) were found to increase BDNF levels as well as improve cognitive functions in rats and humans. BDNF protein and BDNF gene expression (BDNF mRNA) levels in the hippocampus rapidly increased during running exercise and were maintained for several weeks (Cotman, Berchtold, & Christie, 2007). In cross-sectional studies of aged people, serum BDNF levels were significantly associated with cardiorespiratory fitness, psychomotor speed, memory and general cognitive functions, although the findings in one study were confined to a single woman (Komulainen et al., 2008; Swardfager et al., 2011). A randomized control trial by Erickson and colleagues(2011) examined the effects of long-term aerobic exercise on neuro-cognition in elderly adults compared with just stretching. Aerobic exercise was able to effectively reverse hippocampal volume loss and enhanced spatial memory, as well as increase serum BDNF concentrations.

However, a report of an RCT of patients with mild cognitive impairment (MCI) on a six-month high-intensity aerobic exercise programme found no significant increases of serum BDNF in male subjects, but BDNF levels were significantly decreased in female subjects (Baker et al., 2010). Although overwhelming evidence supports BDNF as the most important neutrophic factor in exercise-related enhancement of the brain and improvement of cognition, its accumulation particularly in response to different types, intensities and durations of physical exercise, as well as mechanisms of action across healthy and neuropathological conditions are still poorly understood (Coelho et al., 2013).

Insulin-like growth factor (IGF)

IGF-1 is another known neurotrophic factor associated with aerobic exercise. This growth factor is generated in both the peripheral and central nervous systems, and has a vital role in angiogenesis and neurogenesis induced by aerobic exercise (Ding, Vaynman, Akhavan, Ying, & Gomez-Pinilla, 2006; Trejo, Carro, & Torres-Aleman, 2001). Lower circulating IGF-1 levels observed in older subjects are highly correlated with more severe cognitive impairment, indicating insufficient IGF-1 concentrations could be a biomarker for Alzheimer's Disease (Torres-Aleman, 2008). In animal studies, hippocampal IGF gene expression and IGF plasma concentrations were enhanced by running (Carro, Nunez, Busiguina, & Torres-Aleman, 2000). Trejo and colleagues (2001) suggested that exercise-induced hippocampal neurogenesis could be blocked by blocking the entry of IGF-1 from periphery to the brain. Similar results were observed in exercise-induced hippocampal angiogenesis (Lopez-Lopez, LeRoith, & Torres-Aleman, 2004) and exercise-facilitated brain injury recovery (Carro, Trejo, Busiguina, & Torres-Aleman, 2001).

IGF-1 could also interact with BDNF to modulate exercise-induced synaptic and cognitive plasticity. Ding and colleagues (2006) showed that blocking of the IGF-1 receptors significantly reduced BDNF mRNA and protein levels, suggesting that IGF-1 could partially regulate maturation of the BDNF precursor. Researchers have speculated that attenuation of the increase in BDNF induced by aerobic exercise is potentially due to the down-regulation of IGF-1 with aging (Adlard, Perreau, & Cotman, 2005; Markowska, Mooney, & Sonntag, 1998).

Similar to the inconsistent findings in exercise-induced BDNF, two RCTs did not show elevation of IGF-1 levels after aerobic exercise in young adults. Arikawa and colleagues investigated the changes of IGF binding proteins (IGFBP-1, IGFBP-2, and IGFBP-3) after a 16-week aerobic exercise programme in 319 young females aged 18–30 years. They found a small increase in IGFBP-3 concentrations in the exercise group compared with the controls; no other changes were noted. They concluded that 16-week aerobic exercise had minimum or no effect on IGF proteins (Arikawa, Kurzer, Thomas, & Schmitz, 2010). Schiffer and colleagues examined the effects of moderate strength training and endurance training on plasma concentrations of IGF-1 and BDNF in healthy subjects. IGF-1 basal serum concentration significantly decreased after the interventions in all the groups, but there were no changes in the BDNF concentrations (Schiffer, Schulte, Hollmann, Bloch, & Struder, 2009).

Sympathetic and parasympathetic nervous systems
The main component of yoga involves the practice of deep and slow abdominal breathing fully controlling the rhythm. Slow breathing decreases heart rate, leading to more efficient oxygenation. Mourya and colleagues compared the influences of slow and fast breathing in hypertension and found the slow breathing in yoga brought about a reduction in blood pressure for patients not on any antihypertension medications (Mourya, Mahajan, Singh, & Jain, 2009). They suggested that patients with hypertension suffer from an autonomic dysfunction, an imbalance between the sympathetic and parasympathetic nervous systems. The voluntary control of breathing as practiced in yoga causes alterations in the autonomic system, resulting in improved and balanced autonomic function. Similar hypotheses have also been proposed that yoga may cause a shift toward parasympathetic nervous activity via direct vagal stimulation (Innes, Bourguignon, & Taylor, 2005). Shapiro and colleagues showed that a low-frequency heart rate variability significantly reduced depression following an eight-week yoga programme (Shapiro et al., 2007). Thus, controlled breathing during yoga practice may strengthen parasympathetic nervous activity and attenuate sympathetic nervous activity by modifying cardiac ventricular functioning (Udupa, Madanmohan, Bhavanani, Vijayalakshmi, & Krishnamurthy, 2003; Wein, Andersson, & Erdeus, 2007).

Hypothalamic-pituitary-adrenal (HPA) and regulation of biomarkers
An increasing amount of evidence suggests that certain yoga techniques may improve physical and psychological health through down-regulation of the HPA axis. HPA and the sympathetic nervous system (SNS) are the primary systems that respond to stress, resulting in a series of physiological and psychological effects, such as the release of cortisol and catecholamines (epinephrine and norepinephrine) (Sterling, 2004). This response activates the engagement of energy needed to deal with the stressor through the classic "fight or flight" process. The long-term constant state of hyper-stress leads to repeated and sustained activity of the HPA axis and SNS, which induces dysfunction of the

systems and finally disorders like diabetes, depression, cardiovascular disease and autoimmune disorders (McEwen, 2000).

It has been speculated that yoga may alleviate some psychological symptoms by altering several biological markers and restoring physiological balance. Hypercortisolemia and elevated cortisol levels have been well documented in depression (Burke, Davis, Otte, & Mohr, 2005) and have been observed in some anxiety disorders (Mantella et al., 2008; Schiefelbein, 2006). Several studies have noted that yoga practice significantly reduces salivary cortisol levels both in healthy people (Granath, Ingvarsson, von Thiele, & Lundberg, 2006) and patients with depressive and anxiety disorders (Gangadhar & May, 2000; Michalsen et al., 2005; West, Otte, Geher, Johnson, & Mohr, 2004).

Another promising mechanism suggested by Streeter and colleagues is the elevation of gamma aminobutyric acid (GABA) by yoga. There was a 27% increase in brain GABA levels after an acute yoga session in subjects who regularly practiced yoga, whereas no changes were observed in the control group after a reading session (Streeter et al., 2007). Based on these findings, the authors suggested that yoga might be beneficial for diseases with low GABA levels, such as depression and anxiety disorders.

Serotonin and dopamine systems, two main neurotransmitter systems that show dysfunction in psychiatric disorders, have been proposed as the possible targets for yoga breathing and meditation interventions. During yoga breathing practice where attention is focused on breathing, the oxyhaemoglobin levels were significantly elevated in the anterior prefrontal cortex, and whole-blood serotonin levels were increased associated with increased alpha wave activity measured by electroencephalography (EEG) (Yu et al., 2011). Higher serum dopamine levels were observed in participants performing a moving meditation with natural rhythmic body movements, which was called 'brain wave vibration mind body training'. Furthermore, the increased dopaminergic activity was associated with lower somatic stress and higher positive emotions (Jung et al., 2010). Other hormone chemicals possibly contributing to the beneficial effects of yoga on mental disorders include plasma melatonin and prolactin, whose levels are increased after yoga therapy (Janakiramaiah, 1998; Tooley, Armstrong, Norman, & Sali, 2000).

The mechanisms underlying the improvements in attention and memory by yoga are not completely understood. The positive effects of yoga practice on the psychophysiological parameters related to stress, anxiety and depression could have an indirect benefit on cognitive functions (Rocha et al., 2012). It is well known that memory performance is affected by stress levels (Lupien, Maheu, Tu, Fiocco, & Schramek, 2007). Participants demonstrated an impaired working memory when in a psychosocial stressed state; meanwhile both cortisol levels and sympathetic activity were significantly elevated (Elzinga & Roelofs, 2005). Another study showed a significant correlation between the impaired memory retrieval and the higher cortisol levels in healthy subjects exposed to a social stressor (Buchanan & Tranel, 2008). Similarly, higher anxiety was found to influence the performance of attention-demanding tasks (Fox, 1993). In this respect, the mitigation of negative emotions is considered to mediate the effects of mind-body techniques on cognition in major mental disorders.

Although significant improvements by physical exercise were observed in clinical symptoms, cognitive functions and quality of life of patients with psychosis, the application of different types of exercise in treating the disorder is still in its early stages, and the neurological and biological mechanisms underlying these phenomena are still unknown. The use of exercise therapy in psychosis needs to be further studied to determine which type of exercise is more beneficial, based on the heterogeneity of the disorder, and to understand how the different components of mind-body exercise influence different aspects of the disease.

References

Adlard, P. A., Perreau, V. M., & Cotman, C. W. (2005). The exercise-induced expression of BDNF within the hippocampus varies across life-span. *Neurobiol Aging, 26*(4), 511–520. doi:10.1016/j.neurobiolaging.2004.05.006

Alsina, B., Vu, T., & Cohen-Cory, S. (2001). Visualizing synapse formation in arborizing optic axons in vivo: dynamics and modulation by BDNF. *Nat Neurosci, 4*(11), 1093–1101. doi:10.1038/nn735

Arikawa, A. Y., Kurzer, M. S., Thomas, W., & Schmitz, K. H. (2010). No effect of exercise on insulin-like growth factor-I, insulin, and glucose in young women participating in a 16-week randomized controlled trial. *Cancer Epidemiol Biomarkers Prev, 19*(11), 2987–2990. doi:10.1158/1055-9965.EPI-10-0828

Aron, A. R., Poldrack, R. A., & Wise, S.P. (2009). Cognition: basal ganglia role. In L. R. Squire (Ed.), *Encyclopedia of Neuroscience* (Vol. 2, pp. 1069–1077).

Baker, L. D., Frank, L. L., Foster-Schubert, K., Green, P. S., Wilkinson, C. W., McTiernan, A., . . . Craft, S. (2010). Effects of aerobic exercise on mild cognitive impairment: a controlled trial. *Arch Neurol, 67*(1), 71–79. doi:10.1001/archneurol.2009.307

Balasubramaniam, M., Telles, S., & Doraiswamy, P. M. (2012). Yoga on our minds: a systematic review of yoga for neuropsychiatric disorders. *Front Psychiatry, 3*, 117. doi:10.3389/fpsyt.2012.00117

Barde, Y. A. (1994). Neurotrophins: a family of proteins supporting the survival of neurons. *Prog Clin Biol Res, 390*, 45–56.

Beebe, L. H., Smith, K. D., Roman, M. W., Burk, R. C., McIntyre, K., Dessieux, O. L., . . . Tennison, C. (2013). A Pilot Study Describing Physical Activity in Persons with Schizophrenia Spectrum Disorders (SSDS) after an Exercise Program. *Issues Ment Health Nurs, 34*(4), 214–219. doi:10.3109/01612840.2012.746411

Beebe, L. H., Tian, L., Morris, N., Goodwin, A., Allen, S. S., & Kuldau, J. (2005). Effects of exercise on mental and physical health parameters of persons with schizophrenia. *Issues Ment Health Nurs, 26*(6), 661–676. doi:10.1080/01612840590959551

Behere, R. V., Arasappa, R., Jagannathan, A., Varambally, S., Venkatasubramanian, G., Thirthalli, J., ... Gangadhar, B. N. (2011). Effect of yoga therapy on facial emotion recognition deficits, symptoms and functioning in patients with schizophrenia. *Acta Psychiatr Scand*, 123(2), 147–153. doi:10.1111/j.1600-0447.2010.01605.x

Black, J. E., Isaacs, K. R., Anderson, B. J., Alcantara, A. A., & Greenough, W. T. (1990). Learning causes synaptogenesis, whereas motor activity causes angiogenesis, in cerebellar cortex of adult rats. *Proc Natl Acad Sci U S A*, 87(14), 5568–5572.

Botvinick, M. M., Braver, T. S., Barch, D. M., Carter, C. S., & Cohen, J. D. (2001). Conflict monitoring and cognitive control. *Psychol Rev*, 108(3), 624–652.

Boyke, J., Driemeyer, J., Gaser, C., Buchel, C., & May, A. (2008). Training-induced brain structure changes in the elderly. *J Neurosci*, 28(28), 7031–7035. doi:10.1523/JNEUROSCI.0742-08.2008

Buchanan, T. W., & Tranel, D. (2008). Stress and emotional memory retrieval: effects of sex and cortisol response. *Neurobiol Learn Mem*, 89(2), 134–141. doi:10.1016/j.nlm.2007.07.003

Buchman, A. S., Boyle, P. A., Yu, L., Shah, R. C., Wilson, R. S., & Bennett, D. A. (2012). Total daily physical activity and the risk of AD and cognitive decline in older adults. *Neurology*, 78(17), 1323–1329. doi:10.1212/WNL.0b013e3182535d35

Burke, H. M., Davis, M. C., Otte, C., & Mohr, D. C. (2005). Depression and cortisol responses to psychological stress: a meta-analysis. *Psychoneuroendocrinology*, 30(9), 846–856. doi:10.1016/j.psyneuen.2005.02.010

Carro, E., Nunez, A., Busiguina, S., & Torres-Aleman, I. (2000). Circulating insulin-like growth factor I mediates effects of exercise on the brain. *J Neurosci*, 20(8), 2926–2933.

Carro, E., Trejo, J. L., Busiguina, S., & Torres-Aleman, I. (2001). Circulating insulin-like growth factor I mediates the protective effects of physical exercise against brain insults of different etiology and anatomy. *J Neurosci*, 21(15), 5678–5684.

Casey, B. J., Getz, S., & Galvan, A. (2008). The adolescent brain. *Dev Rev*, 28(1), 62–77. doi:10.1016/j.dr.2007.08.003

Chaddock, L., Erickson, K. I., Prakash, R. S., Kim, J. S., Voss, M. W., Vanpatter, M., ... Kramer, A. F. (2010). A neuroimaging investigation of the association between aerobic fitness, hippocampal volume, and memory performance in preadolescent children. *Brain Res*, 1358, 172–183. doi:10.1016/j.brainres.2010.08.049

Chen, W. C., Chu, H., Lu, R. B., Chou, Y. H., Chen, C. H., Chang, Y. C., ... Chou, K. R. (2009). Efficacy of progressive muscle relaxation training in reducing anxiety in patients with acute schizophrenia. *J Clin Nurs*, 18(15), 2187–2196. doi:10.1111/j.1365-2702.2008.02773.x

Christensen, L. O., Johannsen, P., Sinkjaer, T., Petersen, N., Pyndt, H. S., & Nielsen, J. B. (2000). Cerebral activation during bicycle movements in man. *Exp Brain Res*, 135(1), 66–72.

Clark, P. J., Brzezinska, W. J., Thomas, M. W., Ryzhenko, N. A., Toshkov, S. A., & Rhodes, J. S. (2008). Intact neurogenesis is required for benefits of exercise on spatial memory but not motor performance or contextual fear conditioning in C57BL/6J mice. *Neuroscience*, 155(4), 1048–1058. doi:10.1016/j.neuroscience.2008.06.051

Coelho, F. G., Gobbi, S., Andreatto, C. A., Corazza, D. I., Pedroso, R. V., & Santos-Galduroz, R. F. (2013). Physical exercise modulates peripheral levels of brain-derived neurotrophic factor (BDNF): a systematic review of experimental studies in the elderly. *Arch Gerontol Geriatr*, 56(1), 10–15. doi:10.1016/j.archger.2012.06.003

Cohen, D. L., Wintering, N., Tolles, V., Townsend, R. R., Farrar, J. T., Galantino, M. L., & Newberg, A. B. (2009). Cerebral blood flow effects of yoga training: preliminary evaluation of 4 cases. *J Altern Complement Med*, 15(1), 9–14. doi:10.1089/acm.2008.0008

Colcombe, S. J., Erickson, K. I., Scalf, P. E., Kim, J. S., Prakash, R., McAuley, E., . . . Kramer, A. F. (2006). Aerobic exercise training increases brain volume in aging humans. *J Gerontol A Biol Sci Med Sci*, 61(11), 1166–1170.

Colcombe, S. J., Kramer, A. F., Erickson, K. I., Scalf, P., McAuley, E., Cohen, N. J., . . . Elavsky, S. (2004). Cardiovascular fitness, cortical plasticity, and aging. *Proc Natl Acad Sci U S A*, 101(9), 3316–3321. doi:10.1073/pnas.0400266101

Cotman, C. W., Berchtold, N. C., & Christie, L. A. (2007). Exercise builds brain health: key roles of growth factor cascades and inflammation. *Trends Neurosci*, 30(9), 464–472. doi:10.1016/j.tins.2007.06.011

Creer, D. J., Romberg, C., Saksida, L. M., van Praag, H., & Bussey, T. J. (2010). Running enhances spatial pattern separation in mice. *Proc Natl Acad Sci U S A*, 107(5), 2367–2372. doi:10.1073/pnas.0911725107

De Hert, M., Correll, C. U., Bobes, J., Cetkovich-Bakmas, M., Cohen, D., Asai, I., . . . Leucht, S. (2011). Physical illness in patients with severe mental disorders. I. Prevalence, impact of medications and disparities in health care. *World Psychiatry*, 10(1), 52–77.

De Hert, M., Schreurs, V., Vancampfort, D., & Van Winkel, R. (2009). Metabolic syndrome in people with schizophrenia: a review. *World Psychiatry*, 8(1), 78.

Ding, Q., Vaynman, S., Akhavan, M., Ying, Z., & Gomez-Pinilla, F. (2006). Insulin-like growth factor I interfaces with brain-derived neurotrophic factor-mediated synaptic plasticity to modulate aspects of exercise-induced cognitive function. *Neuroscience*, 140(3), 823–833. doi:10.1016/j.neuroscience.2006.02.084

Duraiswamy, G., Thirthalli, J., Nagendra, H. R., & Gangadhar, B. N. (2007). Yoga therapy as an add-on treatment in the management of patients with schizophrenia—a randomized controlled trial. *Acta Psychiatr Scand*, 116(3), 226–232. doi:10.1111/j.1600-0447.2007.01032.x

Ellis, N., Crone, D., Davey, R., & Grogan, S. (2007). Exercise interventions as an adjunct therapy for psychosis: a critical review. *Br J Clin Psychol*, 46(Pt 1), 95–111.

Elzinga, B. M., & Roelofs, K. (2005). Cortisol-induced impairments of working memory require acute sympathetic activation. *Behav Neurosci*, 119(1), 98–103. doi:10.1037/0735-7044.119.1.98

Engstrom, M., Pihlsgard, J., Lundberg, P., & Soderfeldt, B. (2010). Functional magnetic resonance imaging of hippocampal activation during silent mantra meditation. *J Altern Complement Med*, 16(12), 1253–1258. doi:10.1089/acm.2009.0706

Erickson, K. I., Voss, M. W., Prakash, R. S., Basak, C., Szabo, A., Chaddock, L., . . . Kramer, A. F. (2011). Exercise training increases size of hippocampus and improves memory. *Proc Natl Acad Sci U S A*, 108(7), 3017–3022. doi:10.1073/pnas.1015950108

Evans, K. C., Dougherty, D. D., Schmid, A. M., Scannell, E., McCallister, A., Benson, H., . . . Lazar, S. W. (2009). Modulation of spontaneous breathing via limbic/paralimbic-bulbar circuitry: an event-related fMRI study. *Neuroimage*, 47(3), 961–971. doi:10.1016/j.neuroimage.2009.05.025

Falkai, P., Malchow, B., Wobrock, T., Gruber, O., Schmitt, A., Honer, W. G., . . . Cannon, T. D. (2012). The effect of aerobic exercise on cortical architecture in patients with chronic schizophrenia: a randomized controlled MRI study. *Eur Arch Psychiatry Clin Neurosci*. doi:10.1007/s00406-012-0383-y

Farmer, J., Zhao, X., van Praag, H., Wodtke, K., Gage, F. H., & Christie, B. R. (2004). Effects of voluntary exercise on synaptic plasticity and gene expression in the dentate gyrus of adult male Sprague-Dawley rats in vivo. *Neuroscience*, 124(1), 71–79. doi:10.1016/j.neuroscience.2003.09.029

Ferris, L. T., Williams, J. S., & Shen, C. L. (2007). The effect of acute exercise on serum brain-derived neurotrophic factor levels and cognitive function. *Med Sci Sports Exerc*, 39(4), 728–734. doi:10.1249/mss.0b013e31802f04c7

Fox, E. (1993). Attentional bias in anxiety: selective or not? *Behav Res Ther*, 31(5), 487–493.

Gonzalez-Alonso, J., Dalsgaard, M. K., Osada, T., Volianitis, S., Dawson, E. A., Yoshiga, C. C., & Secher, N. H. (2004). Brain and central haemodynamics and oxygenation during maximal exercise in humans. *J Physiol*, 557(Pt 1), 331–342. doi:10.1113/jphysiol.2004.060574

Graham, K. A., Perkins, D. O., Edwards, L. J., Barrier, R. C., Lieberman, J. A., & Harp, J. B. (2005). Effect of olanzapine on body composition and energy expenditure in adults with first-episode psychosis. *American Journal of Psychiatry*, 162(1), 118–123.

Granath, J., Ingvarsson, S., von Thiele, U., & Lundberg, U. (2006). Stress management: a randomized study of cognitive behavioural therapy and yoga. *Cogn Behav Ther*, 35(1), 3–10. doi:10.1080/16506070500401292

Graybiel, A. M. (2005). The basal ganglia: learning new tricks and loving it. *Curr Opin Neurobiol*, 15(6), 638–644. doi:10.1016/j.conb.2005.10.006

Hawkins, R. C., II, Doell, S. R., Lindseth, P., Jeffers, V., & Skaggs, S. (1980). Anxiety reduction in hospitalized schizophrenics through thermal biofeedback and relaxation training. *Percept Mot Skills*, 51(2), 475–482.

Hillman, C. H., Buck, S. M., Themanson, J. R., Pontifex, M. B., & Castelli, D. M. (2009). Aerobic fitness and cognitive development: Event-related brain potential and task performance indices of executive control in preadolescent children. *Dev Psychol*, 45(1), 114–129. doi:10.1037/a0014437

Hillman, C. H., Castelli, D. M., & Buck, S. M. (2005). Aerobic fitness and neurocognitive function in healthy preadolescent children. *Med Sci Sports Exerc*, 37(11), 1967–1974.

Holley, J., Crone, D., Tyson, P., & Lovell, G. (2011). The effects of physical activity on psychological well-being for those with schizophrenia: A systematic review. *Br J Clin Psychol*, 50(1), 84–105. doi:10.1348/014466510X496220

Holzel, B. K., Ott, U., Gard, T., Hempel, H., Weygandt, M., Morgen, K., & Vaitl, D. (2008). Investigation of mindfulness meditation practitioners with voxel-based morphometry. *Soc Cogn Affect Neurosci*, 3(1), 55–61. doi:10.1093/scan/nsm038

Ide, K., Horn, A., & Secher, N. H. (1999). Cerebral metabolic response to submaximal exercise. *J Appl Physiol*, 87(5), 1604–1608.

Innes, K. E., Bourguignon, C., & Taylor, A. G. (2005). Risk indices associated with the insulin resistance syndrome, cardiovascular disease, and possible protection with yoga: a systematic review. *J Am Board Fam Pract*, 18(6), 491–519.

Isaacs, K. R., Anderson, B. J., Alcantara, A. A., Black, J. E., & Greenough, W. T. (1992). Exercise and the brain: angiogenesis in the adult rat cerebellum after vigorous physical activity and motor skill learning. *J Cereb Blood Flow Metab*, 12(1), 110–119. doi:10.1038/jcbfm.1992.14

Jorgensen, L. G., Perko, M., Hanel, B., Schroeder, T. V., & Secher, N. H. (1992). Middle cerebral artery flow velocity and blood flow during exercise and muscle ischemia in humans. *J Appl Physiol*, 72(3), 1123–1132.

Jung, Y. H., Kang, D. H., Jang, J. H., Park, H. Y., Byun, M. S., Kwon, S. J., . . . Kwon, J. S. (2010). The effects of mind-body training on stress reduction, positive affect, and plasma catecholamines. *Neurosci Lett*, 479(2), 138–142. doi:10.1016/j.neulet.2010.05.048

Kerr, A. L., Steuer, E. L., Pochtarev, V., & Swain, R. A. (2010). Angiogenesis but not neurogenesis is critical for normal learning and memory acquisition. *Neuroscience*, 171(1), 214–226. doi:10.1016/j.neuroscience.2010.08.008

Kilpatrick, L. A., Suyenobu, B. Y., Smith, S. R., Bueller, J. A., Goodman, T., Creswell, J. D., . . . Naliboff, B. D. (2011). Impact of Mindfulness-Based Stress Reduction training on intrinsic brain connectivity. *Neuroimage*, 56(1), 290–298. doi:10.1016/j.neuroimage.2011.02.034

Kleim, J. A., Cooper, N. R., & VandenBerg, P. M. (2002). Exercise induces angiogenesis but does not alter movement representations within rat motor cortex. *Brain Res*, 934(1), 1–6.

Komulainen, P., Pedersen, M., Hanninen, T., Bruunsgaard, H., Lakka, T. A., Kivipelto, M., . . . Rauramaa, R. (2008). BDNF is a novel marker of cognitive function in ageing women: the DR's EXTRA Study. *Neurobiol Learn Mem*, 90(4), 596–603. doi:10.1016/j.nlm.2008.07.014

Laurin, D., Verreault, R., Lindsay, J., MacPherson, K., & Rockwood, K. (2001). Physical activity and risk of cognitive impairment and dementia in elderly persons. *Archives of neurology*, 58(3), 498–504.

Lazar, S. W., Bush, G., Gollub, R. L., Fricchione, G. L., Khalsa, G., & Benson, H. (2000). Functional brain mapping of the relaxation response and meditation. *Neuroreport*, 11(7), 1581–1585.

Lazar, S. W., Kerr, C. E., Wasserman, R. H., Gray, J. R., Greve, D. N., Treadway, M. T., . . . Fischl, B. (2005). Meditation experience is associated with increased cortical thickness. *Neuroreport*, 16(17), 1893–1897.

Lee, E. H., Hui, C. L., Chang, W. C., Chan, S. K., Li, Y. K., Lee, J. T., . . . Chen, E. Y. (2013). Impact of physical activity on functioning of patients with first-episode psychosis—a 6 months prospective longitudinal study. *Schizophr Res*, 150(2–3), 538–541. doi:10.1016/j.schres.2013.08.034

Lee, I.-M., Shiroma, E. J., Lobelo, F., Puska, P., Blair, S. N., & Katzmarzyk, P. T. (2012). Effect of physical inactivity on major non-communicable diseases worldwide: an analysis of burden of disease and life expectancy. *The Lancet*, 380(9838), 219–229.

Leibrock, J., Lottspeich, F., Hohn, A., Hofer, M., Hengerer, B., Masiakowski, P., . . . Barde, Y. A. (1989). Molecular cloning and expression of brain-derived neurotrophic factor. *Nature*, 341(6238), 149–152. doi:10.1038/341149a0

Lindamer, L. A., McKibbin, C., Norman, G. J., Jordan, L., Harrison, K., Abeyesinhe, S., & Patrick, K. (2008). Assessment of physical activity in middle-aged and older adults with schizophrenia. *Schizophr Res*, 104(1–3), 294–301. doi:10.1016/j.schres.2008.04.040

Lohof, A. M., Ip, N. Y., & Poo, M. M. (1993). Potentiation of developing neuromuscular synapses by the neurotrophins NT-3 and BDNF. *Nature*, 363(6427), 350–353. doi:10.1038/363350a0

Lojovich, J. M. (2010). The relationship between aerobic exercise and cognition: is movement medicinal? *J Head Trauma Rehabil*, 25(3), 184–192. doi:10.1097/HTR.0b013e3181dc78cd

Lom, B., & Cohen-Cory, S. (1999). Brain-derived neurotrophic factor differentially regulates retinal ganglion cell dendritic and axonal arborization in vivo. *J Neurosci*, 19(22), 9928–9938.

Lopez-Lopez, C., LeRoith, D., & Torres-Aleman, I. (2004). Insulin-like growth factor I is required for vessel remodeling in the adult brain. *Proc Natl Acad Sci U S A*, 101(26), 9833–9838. doi:10.1073/pnas.0400337101

Luders, E., Toga, A. W., Lepore, N., & Gaser, C. (2009). The underlying anatomical correlates of long-term meditation: larger hippocampal and frontal volumes of gray matter. *Neuroimage*, 45(3), 672–678.

Lupien, S. J., Maheu, F., Tu, M., Fiocco, A., & Schramek, T. E. (2007). The effects of stress and stress hormones on human cognition: Implications for the field of brain and cognition. *Brain Cogn*, 65(3), 209–237. doi:10.1016/j.bandc.2007.02.007

Mantella, R. C., Butters, M. A., Amico, J. A., Mazumdar, S., Rollman, B. L., Begley, A. E., . . . Lenze, E. J. (2008). Salivary cortisol is associated with diagnosis and severity of late-life generalized anxiety disorder. *Psychoneuroendocrinology*, 33(6), 773–781. doi:10.1016/j.psyneuen.2008.03.002

Markowska, A. L., Mooney, M., & Sonntag, W. E. (1998). Insulin-like growth factor-1 ameliorates age-related behavioral deficits. *Neuroscience*, 87(3), 559–569.

Marzolini, S., Jensen, B., Melville, P. (2009). Feasibility and effects of a group-based resistance and aerobic exercise program for individuals with severe schizophrenia: a multidisciplinary approach. *Ment Health Phys Act*, 2, 29–36.

McEwen, B. S. (2000). Allostasis and allostatic load: implications for neuropsychopharmacology. *Neuropsychopharmacology*, 22(2), 108–124. doi:10.1016/S0893-133X(99)00129-3

Michalsen, A., Grossman, P., Acil, A., Langhorst, J., Ludtke, R., Esch, T., ... Dobos, G. J. (2005). Rapid stress reduction and anxiolysis among distressed women as a consequence of a three-month intensive yoga program. *Med Sci Monit*, 11(12), CR555-561.

Mourya, M., Mahajan, A. S., Singh, N. P., & Jain, A. K. (2009). Effect of slow- and fast-breathing exercises on autonomic functions in patients with essential hypertension. *J Altern Complement Med*, 15(7), 711–717. doi:10.1089/acm.2008.0609

Neeper, S. A., Gomez-Pinilla, F., Choi, J., & Cotman, C. W. (1996). Physical activity increases mRNA for brain-derived neurotrophic factor and nerve growth factor in rat brain. *Brain Res*, 726(1–2), 49–56.

O'Callaghan, R. M., Ohle, R., & Kelly, A. M. (2007). The effects of forced exercise on hippocampal plasticity in the rat: a comparison of LTP, spatial- and non-spatial learning. *Behav Brain Res*, 176(2), 362–366. doi:10.1016/j.bbr.2006.10.018

Pagnoni, G., & Cekic, M. (2007). Age effects on gray matter volume and attentional performance in Zen meditation. *Neurobiol Aging*, 28(10), 1623–1627. doi:10.1016/j.neurobiolaging.2007.06.008

Pajonk, F. G., Wobrock, T., Gruber, O., Scherk, H., Berner, D., Kaizl, I., ... Falkai, P. (2010). Hippocampal plasticity in response to exercise in schizophrenia. *Arch Gen Psychiatry*, 67(2), 133–143. doi:10.1001/archgenpsychiatry.2009.193

Pereira, A. C., Huddleston, D. E., Brickman, A. M., Sosunov, A. A., Hen, R., McKhann, G. M., ... Small, S. A. (2007). An in vivo correlate of exercise-induced neurogenesis in the adult dentate gyrus. *Proc Natl Acad Sci U S A*, 104(13), 5638–5643. doi:10.1073/pnas.0611721104

Pharr, O. M., & Coursey, R. D. (1989). The use and utility of EMG biofeedback with chronic schizophrenic patients. *Biofeedback Self Regul*, 14(3), 229–245.

Polich, J. (2007). Updating P300: an integrative theory of P3a and P3b. *Clin Neurophysiol*, 118(10), 2128–2148. doi:10.1016/j.clinph.2007.04.019

Pontifex, M. B., Raine, L. B., Johnson, C. R., Chaddock, L., Voss, M. W., Cohen, N. J., ... Hillman, C. H. (2011). Cardiorespiratory fitness and the flexible modulation of cognitive control in preadolescent children. *J Cogn Neurosci*, 23(6), 1332–1345. doi:10.1162/jocn.2010.21528

Rasmussen, P., Brassard, P., Adser, H., Pedersen, M. V., Leick, L., Hart, E., ... Pilegaard, H. (2009). Evidence for a release of brain-derived neurotrophic factor from the brain during exercise. *Exp Physiol*, 94(10), 1062–1069. doi:10.1113/expphysiol.2009.048512

Redila, V. A., & Christie, B. R. (2006). Exercise-induced changes in dendritic structure and complexity in the adult hippocampal dentate gyrus. *Neuroscience*, 137(4), 1299–1307. doi:10.1016/j.neuroscience.2005.10.050

Rocha, K. K., Ribeiro, A. M., Rocha, K. C., Sousa, M. B., Albuquerque, F. S., Ribeiro, S., & Silva, R. H. (2012). Improvement in physiological and psychological parameters after 6 months of yoga practice. *Conscious Cogn*, 21(2), 843–850. doi:10.1016/j.concog.2012.01.014

Rutherford, L. C., Nelson, S. B., & Turrigiano, G. G. (1998). BDNF has opposite effects on the quantal amplitude of pyramidal neuron and interneuron excitatory synapses. *Neuron*, 21(3), 521–530.

Schiffer, T., Schulte, S., Hollmann, W., Bloch, W., & Struder, H. K. (2009). Effects of strength and endurance training on brain-derived neurotrophic factor and insulin-like growth factor 1 in humans. *Horm Metab Res*, 41(3), 250–254. doi:10.1055/s-0028-1093322

Seil, F. J., & Drake-Baumann, R. (2000). TrkB receptor ligands promote activity-dependent inhibitory synaptogenesis. *J Neurosci*, 20(14), 5367–5373.

Shapiro, D., Cook, I. A., Davydov, D. M., Ottaviani, C., Leuchter, A. F., & Abrams, M. (2007). Yoga as a complementary treatment of depression: effects of traits and moods on treatment outcome. *Evid Based Complement Alternat Med*, 4(4), 493–502. doi:10.1093/ecam/nel114

Shors, T. J., Miesegaes, G., Beylin, A., Zhao, M., Rydel, T., & Gould, E. (2001). Neurogenesis in the adult is involved in the formation of trace memories. *Nature*, 410(6826), 372–376. doi:10.1038/35066584

Shors, T. J., Townsend, D. A., Zhao, M., Kozorovitskiy, Y., & Gould, E. (2002). Neurogenesis may relate to some but not all types of hippocampal-dependent learning. *Hippocampus*, 12(5), 578–584. doi:10.1002/hipo.10103

Spirduso, W. W. (1980). Physical fitness, aging, and psychomotor speed: a review. *J Gerontol*, 35(6), 850–865.

Sterling, P. (2004). Principles of allostasis: optimal design, predictive regulation, pathophysiology, and rational therapeutics. In J. Schulkin (Ed.), *Allostasis, Homeostasis, and the Costs of Physiological Adaptation* (pp. 17–64). Cambridge: Cambridge University Press.

Stranahan, A. M., Khalil, D., & Gould, E. (2007). Running induces widespread structural alterations in the hippocampus and entorhinal cortex. *Hippocampus*, 17(11), 1017–1022. doi:10.1002/hipo.20348

Strassnig, M., Miewald, J., Keshavan, M., & Ganguli, R. (2007). Weight gain in newly diagnosed first-episode psychosis patients and healthy comparisons: one-year analysis. *Schizophr Res*, 93(1), 90–98.

Streeter, C. C., Jensen, J. E., Perlmutter, R. M., Cabral, H. J., Tian, H., Terhune, D. B., ... Renshaw, P. F. (2007). Yoga Asana sessions increase brain

GABA levels: a pilot study. *J Altern Complement Med*, 13(4), 419–426. doi:10.1089/acm.2007.6338

Swain, R. A., Harris, A. B., Wiener, E. C., Dutka, M. V., Morris, H. D., Theien, B. E., ... Greenough, W. T. (2003). Prolonged exercise induces angiogenesis and increases cerebral blood volume in primary motor cortex of the rat. *Neuroscience*, 117(4), 1037–1046.

Swardfager, W., Herrmann, N., Marzolini, S., Saleem, M., Shammi, P., Oh, P. I., ... Lanctot, K. L. (2011). Brain derived neurotrophic factor, cardiopulmonary fitness and cognition in patients with coronary artery disease. *Brain Behav Immun*, 25(6), 1264–1271. doi:10.1016/j.bbi.2011.04.017

Taupin, P. (2006). Neurogenesis in the adult central nervous system. *C R Biol*, 329(7), 465–475. doi:10.1016/j.crvi.2006.04.001

Themanson, J. R., & Hillman, C. H. (2006). Cardiorespiratory fitness and acute aerobic exercise effects on neuroelectric and behavioral measures of action monitoring. *Neuroscience*, 141(2), 757–767. doi:10.1016/j.neuroscience.2006.04.004

Tooley, G. A., Armstrong, S. M., Norman, T. R., & Sali, A. (2000). Acute increases in night-time plasma melatonin levels following a period of meditation. *Biol Psychol*, 53(1), 69–78.

Torres-Aleman, I. (2008). Mouse models of Alzheimer's dementia: current concepts and new trends. *Endocrinology*, 149(12), 5952–5957. doi:10.1210/en.2008-0905

Trejo, J. L., Carro, E., & Torres-Aleman, I. (2001). Circulating insulin-like growth factor I mediates exercise-induced increases in the number of new neurons in the adult hippocampus. *J Neurosci*, 21(5), 1628–1634.

Udupa, K., Madanmohan, Bhavanani, A. B., Vijayalakshmi, P., & Krishnamurthy, N. (2003). Effect of pranayam training on cardiac function in normal young volunteers. *Indian J Physiol Pharmacol*, 47(1), 27–33.

van Praag, H. (2008). Neurogenesis and exercise: past and future directions. *Neuromolecular Med*, 10(2), 128–140. doi:10.1007/s12017-008-8028-z

van Praag, H. (2009). Exercise and the brain: something to chew on. *Trends Neurosci*, 32(5), 283–290. doi:10.1016/j.tins.2008.12.007

van Praag, H., Christie, B. R., Sejnowski, T. J., & Gage, F. H. (1999). Running enhances neurogenesis, learning, and long-term potentiation in mice. *Proc Natl Acad Sci U S A*, 96(23), 13427–13431.

van Praag, H., Kempermann, G., & Gage, F. H. (1999). Running increases cell proliferation and neurogenesis in the adult mouse dentate gyrus. *Nat Neurosci*, 2(3), 266–270. doi:10.1038/6368

van Praag, H., Shubert, T., Zhao, C., & Gage, F. H. (2005). Exercise enhances learning and hippocampal neurogenesis in aged mice. *J Neurosci*, 25(38), 8680–8685. doi:10.1523/JNEUROSCI.1731-05.2005

Vancampfort, D., Correll, C. U., Probst, M., Sienaert, P., Wyckaert, S., De Herdt, A., ... De Hert, M. (2013). A review of physical activity correlates in patients with bipolar disorder. *J Affect Disord*, 145(3), 285–291. doi:10.1016/j.jad.2012.07.020

Vancampfort, D., De Hert, M., Knapen, J., Maurissen, K., Raepsaet, J., Deckx, S., . . . Probst, M. (2011). Effects of progressive muscle relaxation on state anxiety and subjective well-being in people with schizophrenia: a randomized controlled trial. *Clin Rehabil*, 25(6), 567–575. doi:10.1177/0269215510395633

Vancampfort, D., De Hert, M., Knapen, J., Wampers, M., Demunter, H., Deckx, S., . . . Probst, M. (2011). State anxiety, psychological stress and positive well-being responses to yoga and aerobic exercise in people with schizophrenia: a pilot study. *Disabil Rehabil*, 33(8), 684–689. doi:10.3109/09638288.2010.509458

Vancampfort, D., Knapen, J., De Hert, M., . . . Probst, M. (2009). Cardiometabolic effects of physical activity interventions for people with schizophrenia. *Phys Ther Rev.*, 14, 388–398.

Vancampfort, D., Knapen, J., Probst, M., Scheewe, T., Remans, S., & De Hert, M. (2012). A systematic review of correlates of physical activity in patients with schizophrenia. *Acta Psychiatr Scand*, 125(5), 352–362. doi:10.1111/j.1600-0447.2011.01814.x

Vancampfort, D., Vansteelandt, K., Scheewe, T., Probst, M., Knapen, J., De Herdt, A., & De Hert, M. (2012). Yoga in schizophrenia: a systematic review of randomised controlled trials. *Acta Psychiatr Scand*, 126(1), 12–20. doi:10.1111/j.1600-0447.2012.01865.x

Varambally, S., Gangadhar, B. N., Thirthalli, J., Jagannathan, A., Kumar, S., Venkatasubramanian, G., . . . Nagendra, H. R. (2012). Therapeutic efficacy of add-on yogasana intervention in stabilized outpatient schizophrenia: Randomized controlled comparison with exercise and waitlist. *Indian J Psychiatry*, 54(3), 227–232. doi:10.4103/0019-5545.102414

Vestergaard-Poulsen, P., van Beek, M., Skewes, J., Bjarkam, C. R., Stubberup, M., Bertelsen, J., & Roepstorff, A. (2009). Long-term meditation is associated with increased gray matter density in the brain stem. *Neuroreport*, 20(2), 170–174. doi:10.1097/WNR.0b013e328320012a

Visceglia, E., & Lewis, S. (2011). Yoga therapy as an adjunctive treatment for schizophrenia: a randomized, controlled pilot study. *J Altern Complement Med*, 17(7), 601–607. doi:10.1089/acm.2010.0075

Voss, M. W., Prakash, R. S., Erickson, K. I., Basak, C., Chaddock, L., Kim, J. S., . . . Kramer, A. F. (2010). Plasticity of brain networks in a randomized intervention trial of exercise training in older adults. *Front Aging Neurosci*, 2. doi:10.3389/fnagi.2010.00032

Wein, J., Andersson, J. P., & Erdeus, J. (2007). Cardiac and ventilatory responses to apneic exercise. *Eur J Appl Physiol*, 100(6), 637–644. doi:10.1007/s00421-007-0411-1

West, J., Otte, C., Geher, K., Johnson, J., & Mohr, D. C. (2004). Effects of Hatha yoga and African dance on perceived stress, affect, and salivary cortisol. *Ann Behav Med*, 28(2), 114–118. doi:10.1207/s15324796abm2802_6

Weuve, J., Kang, J. H., Manson, J. E., Breteler, M. M., Ware, J. H., & Grodstein, F. (2004). Physical activity, including walking, and cognitive function in older women. *JAMA*, 292(12), 1454–1461.

Yu, X., Fumoto, M., Nakatani, Y., Sekiyama, T., Kikuchi, H., Seki, Y., . . . Arita, H. (2011). Activation of the anterior prefrontal cortex and serotonergic system is associated with improvements in mood and EEG changes induced by Zen meditation practice in novices. *Int J Psychophysiol, 80*(2), 103–111. doi:10.1016/j.ijpsycho.2011.02.004

Zhao, C., Teng, E. M., Summers, R. G., Jr., Ming, G. L., & Gage, F. H. (2006). Distinct morphological stages of dentate granule neuron maturation in the adult mouse hippocampus. *J Neurosci, 26*(1), 3–11. doi:10.1523/JNEUROSCI.3648-05.2006

Zoladz, J. A., Pilc, A., Majerczak, J., Grandys, M., Zapart-Bukowska, J., & Duda, K. (2008). Endurance training increases plasma brain-derived neurotrophic factor concentration in young healthy men. *J Physiol Pharmacol, 59 Suppl* 7, 119–132.

5

Aerobic exercise for people with schizophrenic psychosis

Berend Malchow, Andrea Schmitt and Peter Falkai

Introduction

Schizophrenia is a severe mental disorder that affects humans in young adulthood, often leads to lifelong disability and represents an enormous burden for sufferers and relatives (Murray and Lopez, 1996). Disability is a consequence of cognitive deficits and negative symptoms. Cognitive dysfunction is already present during the prodromal years, before the manifestation of the first episode of schizophrenia, and remains stable over time (Hoff et al., 1999; Hoff et al., 2005). Its core consists mainly of a dysfunction of executive and memory domains, especially verbal memory and cognitive flexibility (Heinrichs and Zakzanis, 1998). The cognitive deficits of schizophrenia patients may contribute to the unfavourable outcome in schizophrenia and may be independent of the long-term course of both positive and negative symptoms (Goff et al., 2011; Green, 1996; Silverstein et al.; 1997). These aforementioned aspects, together with treatment with antipsychotics, may also play a role in schizophrenia patients leading a sedentary, unhealthy lifestyle and therefore experiencing weight gain and increased physical comorbidity and having a significantly reduced life expectancy (Fleischhacker et al., 2008). Both antipsychotic treatment and psychosocial interventions still have limited effects on negative symptoms and cognitive dysfunction (Hasan et al., 2013; Kuipers et al., 2014). Consequently, there is a need for innovative treatment strategies in schizophrenia patients that are effective in the domains of negative symptoms, cognitive dysfunction and social adaptation and hence everyday functioning and quality of life. Current assessments are often based on brief physician-patient contacts and focus on symptoms, but not every day functioning. An understanding of the underlying neurobiology of cognitive dysfunction is important to improve outcome, and parallel investigations of patients and animal models are the best strategy to investigate effects of treatment in the brain.

Physical Exercise Interventions for Mental Health, ed. Linda C. W. Lam and Michelle Riba. Published by Cambridge University Press. © Cambridge University Press 2016.

The hope is that aerobic exercise could play an essential part in regaining regenerative capacities and neuroplasticity in brain regions involved in the pathophysiology of schizophrenia (Hannan, 2014; Falkai et al. 2015).

Neurobiological background

Aerobic exercise has been proposed to influence several biological mechanisms. In mice, voluntary running is known to stimulate adult hippocampal neurogenesis, learning and memory (van Praag et al., 1999; van Praag et al., 2005; Voss et al., 2013); this stimulation also increases exploratory behaviour (Sahay et al., 2011). In healthy humans aerobic exercise was shown to increase hippocampal blood flow (Pereira et al., 2007). In older healthy humans, aerobic exercise was associated with increased hippocampal blood flow, vascularization and hippocampal head volume (Maass et al., 2014). Colcombe and colleagues (2004) reported that exercise not only has a positive influence on the number of synaptic connections, through promoting the development of new neurons, but also increases the cortical capillary blood supply. Aerobic exercise has been associated with increased production of brain neurotrophic factors, like insulin-like growth factor 1 (IGF1), brain-derived neurotrophic factor (BDNF) and vascular endothelial growth factor (VEGF), and increased activity and production of neurotransmitters (serotonin, norepinephrine and dopamine) (Dishman et al., 2006; Raichlen and Polk, 2013; Voss et al., 2013). To date, only a few studies have examined the effects of aerobic exercise in animal models of schizophrenia. For example, in the pharmacological model of MK-801 treatment, enhancement of NMDA receptor expression was reported after treadmill exercise (Park et al., 2014), and behavioural deficits and adult neurogenesis have been shown to be restored in mice after a maternal viral-like infection (Wolf et al., 2011). In humans, one main focus of interventional trials on physical exercise is to evaluate the effects on cognitive performance, individual psychopathology and brain function and structure. In light of the obvious limitations of current pharmacotherapy with antipsychotics and their limited effects on residual symptoms and cognitive deficits, unravelling the neurobiological effects of physical exercise in severe psychiatric diseases may contribute to finding novel treatment strategies, which would presumably act through neuroplastic processes in specific brain regions. In summary, as shown below, aerobic endurance training is known to induce both structural and functional brain changes in schizophrenia patients and animal models for schizophrenia, but it is unknown whether these alterations reflect a reversibility of neurobiological processes directly related to the underlying disease mechanisms. Possible effects of aerobic exercise on neurogenesis, synaptogenesis, prolonged cell survival and changes in vascularization may counteract pathophysiological processes in schizophrenia and influence activity-dependent and experience-dependant structural and functional brain plasticity (Johansen-Berg, 2012; May, 2011).

Aerobic exercise interventions

To date, most exercise intervention studies in schizophrenia have examined the effects of aerobic exercise (Acil et al., 2008; Beebe et al., 2005; Dodd et al., 2011; Falkai et al., 2013; Heggelund et al., 2011; Heggelund et al., 2012; Malchow et al., 2015a; Malchow et al., 2015b; Pajonk et al., 2010), and few studies have combined an aerobic exercise intervention with resistance training (Bredin et al., 2013; Marzolini et al., 2009; Scheewe et al., 2013a; Scheewe et al., 2013b). Studies examining the effects of yoga used a combined aerobic exercise and resistance training programme as a control intervention, the so-called *National Fitness Corps Programme* (Behere et al., 2011; Duraiswamy et al., 2007; Manjunath et al., 2013; Varambally et al., 2012). The use of different types of exercise, such as aerobic exercise, resistance training and relaxation techniques, and selected patient populations makes it difficult to compare exercise interventions. To our knowledge, no study to date has compared purely aerobic exercise directly with resistance training or a sufficient amount of moderate-to-vigorous aerobic exercise directly with yoga. Across studies, not only the duration of the aerobic exercise sessions varies (from 15 minutes up to 135 minutes per week) but also the number of training sessions (from two to five per week). The guidelines of the American College of Sports Medicine (ACSM) recommend 150 minutes of moderate-to-vigorous aerobic exercise split into 3 to 5 sessions of equal duration (Garber et al., 2011), but these recommendations have not sufficiently been addressed in aerobic exercise interventions in schizophrenia.

Impact of aerobic exercise on brain structure

Meta-analyses of structural magnetic resonance imaging (MRI) studies have shown local and overall volume reductions as the most robust findings in schizophrenia patients (Cooper et al., 2014; De Peri et al., 2012; Ellison-Wright and Bullmore, 2010; Haijma et al., 2012; Honea et al., 2005). Hippocampal volumes in particular have been found to be smaller in schizophrenia (Adriano et al., 2012; Steen et al., 2006; Vita and de Peri, 2007); smaller hippocampal volumes seem to be linked to impaired declarative memory function, which is considered a core clinical feature of schizophrenia (Hasan et al., 2013; Tamminga et al., 2010). Furthermore, a growing body of evidence points to the fact that these structural brain changes may be progressive over the course of the illness and may remain regionally distinct (Hulshoff Pol et al., 2002; Mane et al., 2009; Olabi et al., 2011; Vita et al., 2012). However, the underlying pathophysiology of longitudinal alterations is still unclear and may also be related to antipsychotic medication (Lieberman et al., 2005), alcohol and illicit drug use (Van Haren et al., 2012) and differences in activity levels (Vancampfort et al., 2012).

Pajonk and colleagues performed the first MRI study of aerobic exercise in patients with multi-episode schizophrenia (Pajonk et al., 2010). Schizophrenia patients and a control group of healthy individuals performed indoor cycling three times a week for 30 minutes over 3 months; a second, non-exercise control group of schizophrenia patients played table football (known as "foosball" in the USA) at the same frequency and for the same period of time. After indoor cycling, patients showed a hippocampal volume increase of approximately 10%, accompanied by an increase of the N-acetylaspartate/creatinine ratio in MR spectroscopy and an improvement in the short-term memory index (Pajonk et al., 2010). These changes correlated with improved aerobic fitness, indicating for the first time that the hippocampus of schizophrenia patients might be responsive to a plasticity-inducing stimulus. Analysis of cortical surface expansion of patients from the same cohort did not reveal any significant changes in the schizophrenia exercise group com- pared to the healthy participants (Falkai et al., 2013). However, a randomised controlled trial with 63 participants that compared six months of endurance training with occupational therapy in schizophrenia could not replicate these findings (Scheewe et al., 2013b). In a further study, we investigated the effects of a combination of aerobic exercise and targeted computer-assisted cognitive remediation that attempted to mimic an enriched environment intervention and potentially increase the beneficial effect of an aerobic exercise intervention (Malchow et al., 2015a). Twenty multi-episode schizophrenia patients and 21 matched healthy controls underwent the same exercise regimen as described by Pajonk and colleagues (Pajonk et al., 2010); 19 additional schizophrenia patients played table soccer over the same period and served as a schizophrenia control group. In contrast to Pajonk and colleagues (2010) but in line with Scheewe and colleagues (2013b), we did not detect any changes in hippocampal volume or hippocampal subfield volume (Malchow et al., 2015a). When a hypothesis-free longitudinal voxel-based morphometry (VBM) approach was applied to the data, we detected an increase in grey matter volume of the left anterior temporal lobe in the schizophrenia patients after 3 months of endurance training, whereas no such effect was observed in healthy controls or schizophrenia patients playing table soccer. This finding may be relevant for a regenerative process, since the left temporal cortex displays reduced volume in chronic schizophrenia patients (Hazlett et al., 2008). However, the relationship between the observed changes in grey matter volume and the underlying alterations on the cellular or molecular level in schizophrenia patients remains unclear. Until now, only these three neuroima- ging studies with contradictory results have reported the impact of endurance training on brain structure and function in schizophrenia. The total amount of endurance training probably does not play a crucial role in altering brain structure, but rather the frequency and intensity of the training stimulus. In addition, other factors such as the variability of plasticity responses and different sample sizes need to be taken into account when discussing varying results between studies. It is unknown whether the pattern of brain structure changes reported after the aerobic exercise intervention period remains stable in terms of a consolidation process or whether endurance-induced brain volume changes represent only short-term effects that disappear after cessation of the intervention. However, all of these studies support the notion that structural and functional brain changes seen in multi-episode schizophrenia patients may be partially reversible even after a long duration of the disease, which points to disturbed regenerative capacities of the brain rather than a classical degenerative process. The absence of astrogliosis and of neuron loss in post mortem studies of the hippocampus in schizophrenia speaks against a neurodegenerative process (Schmitt et al., 2009).

Impact of aerobic exercise on schizophrenia symptoms

In a clinical study, treadmill walking improved total scores on the Positive and Negative Symptom Scale (PANSS) (Kay et al., 1987) when compared to the waitlist control group, but without reaching statistical significance (Beebe et al., 2005). A significant improvement of overall mental health, measured by the Mental Health Inventory (MHI) (Veit and Ware, 1983), was reported in patients with schizophrenia/schizoaffective disorder who performed a combination of aerobic and resistance exercises compared to the group that received treatment as usual (Marzolini et al., 2009). In the study by Pajonk and colleagues (2010) aerobic exercise reduced schizophrenia symptoms, measured by the PANSS, significantly more than the same amount of table soccer. Likewise, in the study by Scheewe and colleagues (2013a) exercise led to a significant reduction of schizophrenia symptoms, measured by the PANSS, and a significant reduction of depressive symptoms, measured by the Montgomery-Asberg Depression Rating Scale (MADRS; Montgomery and Asberg, 1979). In this study, positive, depressive and emotional symptoms, disorganisation and agitation improved while negative symptoms showed only a trend towards an improvement (Scheewe et al., 2013a). In a comparative study in patients with schizophrenia and depression, negative symptoms in the schizophrenia patients (measured by the PANSS) improved in both the aerobic exercise (circuit training) and the control group (Oertel-Knochel et al., 2014). In our study, we found an improvement in PANSS negative symptoms after three months of endurance training augmented with computer-assisted cognitive remediation (Malchow et al., 2015b). Several studies have reported that yoga improves schizophrenia symptoms more than an aerobic exercise intervention, but in all of these studies the aerobic exercise group served as a control group, and the exercise was only of low intensity (Behere et al., 2011; Duraiswamy et al., 2007; Manjunath et al., 2013; Varambally et al., 2012). A recent systematic review and meta-analysis that included only studies with moderate-to-vigorous amounts of aerobic exercise (as recommended by the American College of Sports Medicine; Garber et al., 2011) reported strong effects of aerobic exercise interventions on reduction of positive and negative symptoms (Firth et al., 2015).

Impact of aerobic exercise on cognition

The above mentioned study in schizophrenia patients by Pajonk and colleagues (2010) found that aerobic endurance training led to improvement in short-term memory (STM) capacity, as measured by the German version of the Rey Auditory Verbal Learning Test (Helmstaedter and Durwen, 1990). However, long-term memory (LTM) capacity and attention span, measured by the Corsi block-tapping test (Milner, 1971), did not change. In contrast, Scheewe and colleagues recorded no alterations in cognition in their studies (personal communication to the authors). A study of aerobic circuit training combined with cognitive remediation showed a significant improvement in schizophrenia patients after exercise therapy in the cognitive domains of processing speed, working memory and visual learning (Oertel-Knochel et al., 2014). When we augmented aerobic exercise with computer-assisted cognitive remediation, we found no improvement in STM when comparing three months of intervention with baseline measures (Malchow et al., 2015b); this finding is in contrast to Pajonk and colleagues (2010).This discrepancy may be due to a larger and more heterogeneous sample in our study. A steady improvement of STM memory capacity only occurred in healthy controls, which may argue for disturbed neuroplasticity in schizophrenia patients. Accordingly, we found no improvement in LTM, cognitive flexibility and task switching, which is in line with previous studies (Malchow et al., 2015b). Interestingly, cognitive flexibility and task switching did improve in the aerobic endurance-training group, but only when scores after three months of training were compared with those after six weeks of training. Because the study did not examine the impact of cognitive remediation or endurance training alone, no final conclusions can be drawn as to exactly which part of the intervention improved cognitive capacity.

Clinical recommendations

On the basis of the aforementioned studies, regular aerobic endurance training can be assumed to significantly improve positive, negative and depressive symptoms in multi-episode schizophrenia when compared with standard care. An improvement of cognitive disabilities is also very likely. Extending aerobic exercise to an enriched-environment experimental setting that combines endurance training with cognitive remediation or cognitive behavioural therapy and relaxation techniques may be beneficial in the treatment of schizophrenia symptoms. Endurance training with exercise bicycles (ergometers) is a cheap and safe method, and easy to implement in a multimodal treatment concept. In addition, it should be noted that regular endurance training may have positive effects on the course of metabolic syndrome, which is common in schizophrenia patients (Bredin et al., 2013; Heggelund et al., 2011; Scheewe et al., 2013a). One can expect to see benefits in inpatients, patients at day-care clinics and outpatients. Because humans take at least six weeks to adapt to a new endurance-training stimulus, longer treatment periods are recommended. Additionally, before starting a training programme patients' physical health should be carefully assessed (e.g., electrocardiogram (ECG), blood pressure, blood parameters) (Hottenrott and Neumann, 2010). Group sessions are recommended to improve compliance;

sessions should be supervised to maintain attendance rates and carefully monitor patients' exhaustion levels. Cycling on an exercise bicycle is a very joint-friendly kind of aerobic exercise, because the participants do not have to carry their own weight. The circular movement of the legs is easy and may also have a relaxing effect, because of the rhythmic repetitions. Nevertheless, as part of a long-term exercise therapy regimen, other aerobic exercises such as running on a treadmill may also appeal to patients and help to avoid monotonous training stimuli.

Future research strategies

The effects of aerobic exercise in recent-onset schizophrenia patients or people at high risk of developing a psychotic disorder are unknown, and a larger controlled study with an extended exercise period of up to six months that includes gradual increases in treatment intensity is needed to establish a validated protocol for the treatment of negative symptoms and cognitive dysfunction through aerobic exercise in this population. Moreover, duration and intensity of the aerobic exercise intervention should be studied in more detail. Additionally, it is unknown how long the exercise-dependent effects last after completion of the intervention. The underlying mechanisms of exercise-dependent alterations in brain structure and function, and the factors that may predict treatment response still remain largely unknown and should be studied in larger cohorts of schizophrenia patients and healthy controls. We detected stronger effects of aerobic exercise on physical fitness in healthy men with schizophrenia than in women. Consequently, sex-related treatment effects should be investigated in more detail; on the basis of our findings (Malchow et al., 2015b), men can be assumed to benefit to a larger extent than women from an endurance training intervention.

There is still a need for innovative treatment strategies for schizophrenia that are effective in the domains of cognitive dysfunction and negative symptoms and in everyday functioning and subjective well-being. The use of aerobic exercise in multi-modal treatment approaches may lessen the burden of disease in this severely affected patient group.

References

Acil, A. A., Dogan, S. & Dogan, O. 2008. The effects of physical exercises to mental state and quality of life in patients with schizophrenia. *J Psychiatr Ment Health Nurs*, 15, 808–15.

Adriano, F., Caltagirone, C. & Spalletta, G. 2012. Hippocampal volume reduction in first-episode and chronic schizophrenia: a review and meta-analysis. *Neuroscientist*, 18, 180–200.

Behere, R. V., Arasappa, R., Jagannathan, A., Varambally, S., Venkatasubramanian, G., Thirthalli, J., Subbakrishna, D. K., Nagendra, H. R. & Gangadhar, B. N. 2011.

Effect of yoga therapy on facial emotion recognition deficits, symptoms and functioning in patients with schizophrenia. *Acta psychiatrica Scandinavica*, 123, 147–53.

Bredin, S. S., Warburton, D. E. & Lang, D. J. 2013. The health benefits and challenges of exercise training in persons living with schizophrenia: a pilot study. *Brain Sci*, 3, 821–48.

Colcombe, S. J., Kramer, A. F., Mcauley, E., Erickson, K. I. & Scalf, P. 2004. Neurocognitive aging and cardiovascular fitness: recent findings and future directions. *J Mol Neurosci*, 24, 9–14.

Cooper, D., Barker, V., Radua, J., Fusar-Poli, P. & Lawrie, S. M. 2014. Multimodal voxel-based meta-analysis of structural and functional magnetic resonance imaging studies in those at elevated genetic risk of developing schizophrenia. *Psychiatry Res*, 221, 69–77.

De Peri, L., Crescini, A., Deste, G., Fusar-Poli, P., Sacchetti, E. & Vita, A. 2012. Brain structural abnormalities at the onset of schizophrenia and bipolar disorder: a meta-analysis of controlled magnetic resonance imaging studies. *Current pharmaceutical design*, 18, 486–94.

Dishman, R. K., Berthoud, H. R., Booth, F. W., Cotman, C. W., Edgerton, V. R., Fleshner, M. R., Gandevia, S. C., Gomez-Pinilla, F., Greenwood, B. N., Hillman, C. H., Kramer, A. F., Levin, B. E., Moran, T. H., Russo-Neustadt, A. A., Salamone, J. D., Van Hoomissen, J. D., Wade, C. E., York, D. A. & Zigmond, M. J. 2006. Neurobiology of exercise. *Obesity (Silver Spring)*, 14, 345–56.

Dodd, K. J., Duffy, S., Stewart, J. A., Impey, J. & Taylor, N. 2011. A small group aerobic exercise programme that reduces body weight is feasible in adults with severe chronic schizophrenia: a pilot study. *Disabil Rehabil*, 33, 1222–9.

Duraiswamy, G., Thirthalli, J., Nagendra, H. R. & Gangadhar, B. N. 2007. Yoga therapy as an add-on treatment in the management of patients with schizo-phrenia—a randomized controlled trial. *Acta psychiatrica Scandinavica*, 116, 226–32.

Ellison-Wright, I. & Bullmore, E. 2010. Anatomy of bipolar disorder and schizo-phrenia: a meta-analysis. *Schizophrenia research*, 117, 1–12.

Falkai, P., Malchow, B., Wobrock, T., Gruber, O., Schmitt, A., Honer, W. G., Pajonk, F. G., Sun, F. & Cannon, T. D. 2013. The effect of aerobic exercise on cortical architecture in patients with chronic schizophrenia: a randomized controlled MRI study. *Eur Arch Psychiatry Clin Neurosci*, 263, 469–73.

Falkai, P., Rossner, M. J., Schulze, T. G., Hasan, A., Brzózka, M. M., Malchow, B., Honer W. G., Schmitt, A. 2015. Kraepelin revisited: schizophrenia from degeneration to failed regeneration. *Mol Psychiatry*, 20(6), 671-6.

Firth, J., Cotter, J., Elliott, R., French, P. & Yung, A. R. 2015. A systematic review and meta-analysis of exercise interventions in schizophrenia patients. *Psychol Med*, 1–19.

Fleischhacker, W. W., Cetkovich-Bakmas, M., De Hert, M., Hennekens, C. H., Lambert, M., Leucht, S., Maj, M., Mcintyre, R. S., Naber, D., Newcomer, J. W., Olfson, M., Osby, U., Sartorius, N. & Lieberman, J. A. 2008. Comorbid somatic illnesses in patients with severe mental disorders: clinical, policy, and research challenges. *J Clin Psychiatry*, 69, 514–9.

Garber, C. E., Blissmer, B., Deschenes, M. R., Franklin, B. A., Lamonte, M. J., Lee, I. M., Nieman, D. C. & Swain, D. P. 2011. American College of Sports Medicine position stand. Quantity and quality of exercise for developing and maintaining cardiorespiratory, musculoskeletal, and neuromotor fitness in apparently healthy adults: guidance for prescribing exercise. *Med Sci Sports Exerc*, 43, 1334–59.

Goff, D. C., Hill, M. & Barch, D. 2011. The treatment of cognitive impairment in schizophrenia. *Pharmacol Biochem Behav*, 99, 245–53.

Green, M. F. 1996. What are the functional consequences of neurocognitive deficits in schizophrenia? *The American Journal of Psychiatry*, 153, 321–30.

Haijma, S. V., Van Haren, N., Cahn, W., Koolschijn, P. C., Hulshoff Pol, H. E. & Kahn, R. S. 2012. Brain Volumes in Schizophrenia: a Meta-Analysis in Over 18 000 Subjects. *Schizophrenia bulletin*, 39(5):1129–38.

Hannan, A. J. 2014. Environmental enrichment and brain repair: harnessing the therapeutic effects of cognitive stimulation and physical activity to enhance experience-dependent plasticity. *Neuropathol Appl Neurobiol*, 40, 13–25.

Hasan, A., Falkai, P., Wobrock, T., Lieberman, J., Glenthoj, B., Gattaz, W. F., Thibaut, F., Moller, H. J. & WFSBP Task force on Treatment Guidelines for Schizophrenia 2013. World Federation of Societies of Biological Psychiatry (WFSBP) guidelines for biological treatment of schizophrenia, part 2: update 2012 on the long-term treatment of schizophrenia and management of antipsychotic-induced side effects. *World J Biol Psychiatry*, 14, 2–44.

Hazlett, E. A., Buchsbaum, M. S., Haznedar, M. M., Newmark, R., Goldstein, K. E., Zelmanova, Y., Glanton, C. F., Torosjan, Y., New, A. S., Lo, J. N., Mitropoulou, V. & Siever, L. J. 2008. Cortical gray and white matter volume in unmedicated schizotypal and schizophrenia patients. *Schizophr Res*, 101, 111–23.

Heggelund, J., Morken, G., Helgerud, J., Nilsberg, G. E. & Hoff, J. 2012. Therapeutic effects of maximal strength training on walking efficiency in patients with schizophrenia—a pilot study. *BMC Res Notes*, 5, 344.

Heggelund, J., Nilsberg, G. E., Hoff, J., Morken, G. & Helgerud, J. 2011. Effects of high aerobic intensity training in patients with schizophrenia: a controlled trial. *Nord J Psychiatry*, 65, 269–75.

Heinrichs, R. W. & Zakzanis, K. K. 1998. Neurocognitive deficit in schizophrenia: a quantitative review of the evidence. *Neuropsychology*, 12, 426–45.

Helmstaedter, C. & Durwen, H. F. 1990. The Verbal Learning and Retention Test. A useful and differentiated tool in evaluating verbal memory performance. *Schweiz Arch Neurol Psychiatr*, 141, 21–30.

Hoff, A. L., Sakuma, M., Wieneke, M., Horon, R., Kushner, M. & Delisi, L. E. 1999. Longitudinal neuropsychological follow-up study of patients with first-episode schizophrenia. *American Journal of Psychiatry*, 156, 1336–41.

Hoff, A. L., Svetina, C., Shields, G., Stewart, J. & Delisi, L. E. 2005. Ten year longitudinal study of neuropsychological functioning subsequent to a first episode of schizophrenia. *Schizophrenia research*, 78, 27–34.

Honea, R., Crow, T. J., Passingham, D. & Mackay, C. E. 2005. Regional deficits in brain volume in schizophrenia: a meta-analysis of voxel-based morphometry studies. *American Journal of Psychiatry*, 162, 2233–45.

Hottenrott, K. & Neumann, G. 2010. *Methods of endurance training*. Schorndorf: Verlag Karl Hofmann.

Hulshoff Pol, H. E., Schnack, H. G., Bertens, M. G., Van Haren, N. E., Van Der Tweel, I., Staal, W. G., Baare, W. F. & Kahn, R. S. 2002. Volume changes in gray matter in patients with schizophrenia. *American Journal of Psychiatry*, 159, 244–50.

Johansen-Berg, H. 2012. The future of functionally-related structural change assessment. *Neuroimage*, 62, 1293–8.

Kay, S. R., Fiszbein, A. & Opler, L. A. 1987. The positive and negative syndrome scale (PANSS) for schizophrenia. *Schizophrenia bulletin*, 13, 261–76.

Kuipers, E., Yesufu-Udechuku, A., Taylor, C. & Kendall, T. 2014. Management of psychosis and schizophrenia in adults: summary of updated NICE guidance. *BMJ*, 348, g1173.

Lieberman, J. A., Tollefson, G. D., Charles, C., Zipursky, R., Sharma, T., Kahn, R. S., Keefe, R. S., Green, A. I., Gur, R. E., Mcevoy, J., Perkins, D., Hamer, R. M., Gu, H. & Tohen, M. 2005. Antipsychotic drug effects on brain morphology in first-episode psychosis. *Archives of general psychiatry*, 62, 361–70.

Maass, A., Duzel, S., Goerke, M., Becke, A., Sobieray, U., Neumann, K., Lovden, M., Lindenberger, U., Backman, L., Braun-Dullaeus, R., Ahrens, D., Heinze, H. J., Muller, N. G. & Duzel, E. 2014. Vascular hippocampal plasticity after aerobic exercise in older adults. *Mol Psychiatry*, 20(5), 585–93.

Malchow, B., Keeser, D., Keller, K., Hasan, A., Rauchmann, B. S., Kimura, H., Schneider-Axmann, T., Dechent, P., Gruber, O., Ertl-Wagner, B., Honer, W. G., Hillmer-Vogel, U., Schmitt, A., Wobrock, T., Niklas, A. & Falkai, P. 2015a. Effects of endurance training on brain structures in chronic schizophrenia patients and healthy controls. *Schizophr Res.*, DOI: http://dx.doi.org/10.1016/j.schres.2015.01.005.

Malchow, B., Keller-Varady, K., Hasan, A., Dörfler, S., Schneider-Axmann, T., Hillmer-Vogel, U., Honer, W. G., Schulze, T. G., Niklas, A., Wobrock, T., Schmitt, A. & Falkai, P. 2015b. Effects of endurance training combined with cognitive remediation on everyday functioning, symptoms and cognition in multi-episode schizophrenia patients. *Schizophrenia Bulletin*, 41(4), 847-58.

Mane, A., Falcon, C., Mateos, J. J., Fernandez-Egea, E., Horga, G., Lomena, F., Bargallo, N., Prats-Galino, A., Bernardo, M. & Parellada, E. 2009. Progressive gray matter changes in first episode schizophrenia: a 4-year longitudinal magnetic resonance study using VBM. *Schizophr Res*, 114, 136–43.

Manjunath, R. B., Varambally, S., Thirthalli, J., Basavaraddi, I. V. & Gangadhar, B. N. 2013. Efficacy of yoga as an add-on treatment for in-patients with functional psychotic disorder. *Indian J Psychiatry*, 55, S374-8.

Marzolini, S., Jensen, B. & Melville, P. 2009. Feasibility and effects of a group-based resistance and aerobic exercise program for individuals with severe schizophrenia: a multidisciplinary approach. *Mental Health and Physical Activity*, 2, 29–36.

May, A. 2011. Experience-dependent structural plasticity in the adult human brain. *Trends Cogn Sci*, 15, 475–82.

Milner, B. 1971. Interhemispheric differences in the localization of psychological processes in man. *Br Med Bull*, 27, 272–7.

Montgomery, S. A. & Asberg, M. 1979. A new depression scale designed to be sensitive to change. *British Journal of Psychiatry*, 134, 382–9.

Murray, C. J. & Lopez, A. D. 1996. Evidence-based health policy—lessons from the Global Burden of Disease Study. *Science*, 274, 740–3.

Oertel-Knochel, V., Mehler, P., Thiel, C., Steinbrecher, K., Malchow, B., Tesky, V., Ademmer, K., Prvulovic, D., Banzer, W., Zopf, Y., Schmitt, A. & Hansel, F. 2014. Effects of aerobic exercise on cognitive performance and individual psychopathology in depressive and schizophrenia patients. *Eur Arch Psychiatry Clin Neurosci*, 264(7), 589–604.

Olabi, B., Ellison-Wright, I., Mcintosh, A. M., Wood, S. J., Bullmore, E. & Lawrie, S. M. 2011. Are there progressive brain changes in schizophrenia? A meta-analysis of structural magnetic resonance imaging studies. *Biol Psychiatry*, 70, 88–96.

Pajonk, F. G., Wobrock, T., Gruber, O., Scherk, H., Berner, D., Kaizl, I., Kierer, A., Muller, S., Oest, M., Meyer, T., Backens, M., Schneider-Axmann, T., Thornton, A. E., Honer, W. G. & Falkai, P. 2010. Hippocampal plasticity in response to exercise in schizophrenia. *Archives of general psychiatry*, 67, 133–43.

Park, J. K., Lee, S. J. & Kim, T. W. 2014. Treadmill exercise enhances NMDA receptor expression in schizophrenia mice. *J Exerc Rehabil*, 10, 15–21.

Pereira, A. C., Huddleston, D. E., Brickman, A. M., Sosunov, A. A., Hen, R., Mckhann, G. M., Sloan, R., Gage, F. H., Brown, T. R. & Small, S. A. 2007. An in vivo correlate of exercise-induced neurogenesis in the adult dentate gyrus. *Proceedings of the National Academy of Sciences of the United States of America*, 104, 5638–43.

Raichlen, D. A. & Polk, J. D. 2013. Linking brains and brawn: exercise and the evolution of human neurobiology. *Proc Biol Sci*, 280, 20122250.

Sahay, A., Scobie, K. N., Hill, A. S., O'Carroll, C. M., Kheirbek, M. A., Burghardt, N. S., Fenton, A. A., Dranovsky, A. & Hen, R. 2011. Increasing adult hippocampal neurogenesis is sufficient to improve pattern separation. *Nature*, 472, 466–70.

Scheewe, T. W., Backx, F. J., Takken, T., Jorg, F., Van Strater, A. C., Kroes, A. G., Kahn, R. S. & Cahn, W. 2013a. Exercise therapy improves mental and physical health in schizophrenia: a randomised controlled trial. *Acta Psychiatr Scand*, 127, 464–73.

Scheewe, T. W., Van Haren, N. E., Sarkisyan, G., Schnack, H. G., Brouwer, R. M., De Glint, M., Hulshoff Pol, H. E., Backx, F. J., Kahn, R. S. & Cahn, W. 2013b. Exercise therapy, cardiorespiratory fitness and their effect on brain volumes: a randomised controlled trial in patients with schizophrenia and healthy controls. *Eur Neuropsychopharmacol*, 23, 675–85.

Schmitt, A., Steyskal, C., Bernstein, H. G., Schneider-Axmann, T., Parlapani, E., Schaeffer, E. L., Gattaz, W. F., Bogerts, B., Schmitz, C. & Falkai, P. 2009. Stereologic investigation of the posterior part of the hippocampus in schizophrenia. *Acta neuropathologica*, 117, 395–407.

Silverstein, M. L., Harrow, M., Mavrolefteros, G. & Close, D. 1997. Neuropsychological dysfunction and clinical outcome in psychiatric disorders: a two-year follow-up study. *J Nerv Ment Dis*, 185, 722–9.

Steen, R. G., Mull, C., Mcclure, R., Hamer, R. M. & Lieberman, J. A. 2006. Brain volume in first-episode schizophrenia: systematic review and meta-analysis of magnetic resonance imaging studies. *British Journal of Psychiatry*, 188, 510–8.

Tamminga, C. A., Stan, A. D. & Wagner, A. D. 2010. The hippocampal formation in schizophrenia. *Am J Psychiatry*, 167, 1178–93.

Van Haren, N. E., Cahn, W., Hulshoff Pol, H. E. & Kahn, R. S. 2012. Confounders of excessive brain volume loss in schizophrenia. *Neuroscience and biobehavioral reviews*, 37(10 Pt 1), 2418–23.

Van Praag, H., Kempermann, G. & Gage, F. H. 1999. Running increases cell proliferation and neurogenesis in the adult mouse dentate gyrus. *Nature neuroscience*, 2, 266–70.

Van Praag, H., Shubert, T., Zhao, C. & Gage, F. H. 2005. Exercise enhances learning and hippocampal neurogenesis in aged mice. *Journal of Neuroscience*, 25, 8680–5.

Vancampfort, D., Knapen, J., Probst, M., Scheewe, T., Remans, S. & De Hert, M. 2012. A systematic review of correlates of physical activity in patients with schizophrenia. *Acta psychiatrica Scandinavica*, 125, 352–62.

Varambally, S., Gangadhar, B. N., Thirthalli, J., Jagannathan, A., Kumar, S., Venkatasubramanian, G., Muralidhar, D., Subbakrishna, D. K. & Nagendra, H. R. 2012. Therapeutic efficacy of add-on yogasana intervention in stabilized outpatient schizophrenia: randomized controlled comparison with exercise and waitlist. *Indian J Psychiatry*, 54, 227–32.

Veit, C. T. & Ware, J. E. 1983. The structure of psychological distress and well-being in general populations. *J Consult Clin Psychol*, 51, 730–742.

Vita, A. & De Peri, L. 2007. Hippocampal and amygdala volume reductions in first-episode schizophrenia. *British Journal of Psychiatry*, 190, 271.

Vita, A., De Peri, L., Deste, G. & Sacchetti, E. 2012. Progressive loss of cortical gray matter in schizophrenia: a meta-analysis and meta-regression of longitudinal MRI studies. *Transl Psychiatry*, 2, e190.

Voss, M. W., Vivar, C., Kramer, A. F. & Van Praag, H. 2013. Bridging animal and human models of exercise-induced brain plasticity. *Trends Cogn Sci*, 17, 525–44.

Wolf, S. A., Melnik, A. & Kempermann, G. 2011. Physical exercise increases adult neurogenesis and telomerase activity, and improves behavioral deficits in a mouse model of schizophrenia. *Brain Behav Immun*, 25, 971–80.

6

Physical exercise to calm your 'nerves'

Linda C. W. Lam, Arthur D. P. Mak and Sing Lee

Anxiety: a psycho-biological manifestation of stress

Anxiety is a psycho-biological response to stress and prepares a person to remain alert and watchful. It is not uncommon for a person to experience anxiety symptoms in face of stressful life events. An appropriate level of anxiety constitutes the psychological preparedness essential for adaptation of environmental stimuli. However, great variations in individual susceptibility also mean that some people may experience intense anxiety grossly in excess of the reactions expected for situations which many others do not find threatening or worrying.

In people with anxiety symptoms severe enough to cause disturbances in everyday functioning, the diagnoses of anxiety disorders should be considered. Anxiety disorders, such as Generalized Anxiety Disorders (GAD) and Panic Disorder, are highly prevalent conditions in the community. Studies have reported that about 10% of the general population may be suffering from different forms of anxiety disorders, which are also among the commonest illnesses presenting to primary care (Kessler et al., 2010; Kroenke et al., 2007). The psychosocial impairment associated with anxiety disorders has been less recognized than that of Major Depressive Disorder (MDD). While it is generally assumed that anxiety is a more benign condition compared to mood disorders, recent studies attest to both the chronicity of anxiety disorders and their substantial impact on a person's quality of life. These are well illustrated in Generalized Anxiety Disorder and Panic Disorder, which are the two commonest anxiety disorders (Kessler et al., 2010). Accordingly, the *Diagnostic and Statistical Manual for Mental Disorder*, 5th edition (DSM-5) highlights, in the case of the diagnosis of Generalized Anxiety Disorder (GAD), the core feature of apprehensive anticipation when excessive and uncontrollable worries would be present for most of the day for at least six months. Such worries lead to clinically significant

Physical Exercise Interventions for Mental Health, ed. Linda C. W. Lam and Michelle Riba. Published by Cambridge University Press. © Cambridge University Press 2016.

Table 6.1 *Clinical features of Generalized Anxiety & Panic Disorders (Adapted from DSM-5 criteria)*

	Generalized Anxiety Disorder	Panic Disorder
Apprehensive Expectations	Excessive worries and anxiety occurring on most days	Recurrent unexpected attacks. Abrupt surge of irrational fear or intense discomfort
Duration	At least 6 months	At least one attack followed by one month of anticipatory fear of attacks
Self-control and functioning	Difficulty in self-control with disturbances in daily functioning	Maladaptive behavior
Symptoms	Three or more	Four or more during attacks
	Restlessness or feeling keyed up, on edge	Palpitation, pounding heart, accelerated heart rate
	Easily fatigued	Sweating
	Difficulty concentrating	Trembling or shaking
	Irritability	Sensation of shortness of breath
	Muscle tension	Feeling of choking
	Sleep disturbances	Chest discomfort
		Nausea or abdominal distress
		Feeling dizzy
		Chill or heat
		Numbness or tingling
		Derealization or depersonalization
		Fear of getting crazy
		Fear of dying

impairment in affected individuals. In Panic Disorder, episodic attacks of intense dreadful feelings with prominent physiological symptoms such as palpitation, chest tightness and abdominal discomfort are characteristic (Table 6.1) (APA, 2013).

Anxiety disorders are characterized not only by prominent psychological worry and fear but also by distressing physical symptoms. Although the latter are often not required for diagnosis in the DSM-5 conceptualization of anxiety disorders, they are clinically relevant and highly correlated with the symptoms of co-existing medical conditions, such as gastrointestinal, cardiac and musculoskeletal disorders. These physical symptoms may create a vicious spiral that amplifies the illness anxiety and health-related behaviours of affected individuals (Lee et al., 2014).

Treatment is frequently suboptimal

Although anxiety disorders are highly prevalent, their treatment has been far from satisfactory. For individuals with mild and uncomplicated anxiety disorders, general recommendations frequently include self-help and psychoeducation on stress management in combination with watchful monitoring. In patients with more significant anxiety symptoms and psychosocial impairment, more structured psychosocial interventions such as progressive relaxation, physical exercise and cognitive behavioural therapy are generally recommended treatment options. In people suffering from severe symptoms that are refractory to psychosocial

Table 6.2 *Principles of Management for Anxiety Disorders (adapted from Nice guidelines, 2013)*

	Mild	Moderate (with psychosocial impairments)	Severe (complex disorders with comorbidity)
Observation and monitoring	Monitoring and observation	–	
Psychosocial interventions	Counseling Self-help Psychoeducation Physical exercise	Group therapy, cognitive behavioural therapy, relaxation Physical exercise	Group therapy Cognitive behavioural therapy, relaxation Physical exercise
Pharmacotherapy	Not recommended	Short-term benzodiazepine Selective serotonin reuptake inhibitors Pregabalin	Short-term benzodiazepine Selective serotonin reuptake inhibitors Pregabalin

interventions, pharmacological interventions include selective serotonin reuptake inhibitors, short-term benzodiazepines or pregabalin (Farach et al., 2012). However, drug treatments are limited by side effects and possible risks of dependence. Also, these disorders tend to run a chronic course and complete remission of anxiety symptoms following drug therapy is uncommon (Table 6.2).

Physical exercise may reduce anxiety

Risk factors for anxiety disorders are complex in origin and vary across affected individuals. Apart from genetic factors, personality predisposition, childhood adversity, psychosocial situations, physical illness burden and life events have all been associated with the development and persistence of anxiety disorders. Physical exercise could form an important part of a multi-dimensional management approach that incorporates the empowerment of self-mastery in developing internal strategies to regulate different symptom dimensions in reaction to stressful situations in life.

There have been numerous studies to suggest that physical exercise may exert a beneficial effect on anxiety symptoms. Earlier reports have suggested that physical exercise, both aerobic and non-aerobic forms of exercise, may exert an acute anxiolytic effect and be developed into potential treatment modalities in both *subthreshold anxiety* and clinical disorders (Byrne & Byrne, 1993; Martinsen et al., 1989; Petruzzello et al., 1991; Tkachuk & Martin, 1999).

Relationship of physical activity with anxiety symptoms in the general population

Epidemiological studies have reported a negative association between physical activity and anxiety levels in the general population. A higher level of physical exercise is associated with lower anxiety scores. In the National Comorbidity Survey (n = 8098) in the United States, 60.3% of participants reported regular physical activity, which was associated with significantly reduced prevalence for current major depressive and anxiety disorders. The association between regular physical activity and prevalence of major depression (OR = 0.75(0.6, 0.94)), panic attacks (OR = 0.73(0.56, 0.96)), social phobia (OR = 0.65(0.53, 0.8)), specific phobia (OR = 0.78(0.63, 0.97)) persisted after adjustment with sociodemographic characteristics, self-report physical illness and current mental disorders (Goodwin, 2003). In the Netherlands Twin Registry, when twins and families participated in a population-based survey (n = 19,288), regular exercise participation was also significantly associated with lower prevalence of anxiety and depression (De Moor et al., 2006). When analysed against genetic factors, this population-based cohort also found physical exercise to be associated with reduced anxiety symptoms independent of genetic risk, but a causal relationship could not be established (De Moor et al., 2008).

The benefits of physical activity are certainly not confined to mental health. Reviews of cross-sectional and prospective studies, as well as randomized controlled trials, suggested, however, that regular physical activities were associated with better health outcomes in both physical and mental conditions (Barbour et al., 2007; Penedo & Dahn, 2005). It is also plausible, therefore that physical activity benefited mental health in part due to its to its benefit on physical health, as the physical conditions studied, including obesity, arthritis, sexual dysfunction, cancer, and coronary heart disease, all have bi-directional associations with mental health outcomes.

Physical exercise for anxiety sensitivity

Anxiety sensitivity is an enduring fear of anxiety-related situations, frequently associated with the belief that anxiety symptoms were harmful to body and health. It is recognized as a character predisposition in which the person is prone to developing both physiological and psychological symptoms of anxiety, particularly panic disorders.

In studies examining people with anxiety sensitivity, experimental paradigms were used to examine the effects of aerobic exercise in alleviating anxiety symptoms and fear (Smits et al., 2008). In a study that examined effects of six sessions of high- (n = 29) versus low-intensity (n = 25) aerobic exercise on anxiety sensitivity, both types of exercise reduced self-ratings of anxiety sensitivity. High-intensity exercise was associated with a faster drop in general anxiety measures with more treatment responders (Broman-Fulks et al., 2004). In another 6-week randomized controlled intervention of brief aerobic exercise in 24 participants with high anxiety sensitivity scores, exercise intervention was associated with a significant reduction of anxiety sensitivity as compared to controls (Broman-Fulks & Storey, 2008).

Physical exercise for anxiety disorders

Progressive muscle relaxation and breathing exercise are recommended interventions for mild to moderate anxiety. However, despite the long history of studies in this area, the therapeutic effects of these interventions on anxiety have not been fully evaluated (Burbach, 1997). Although breathing and relaxation techniques are commonly used in clinical settings, most research has focused on aerobic exercise.

Relatively few studies have adopted a structured approach to examining specific physical exercise interventions, either as sole or adjunctive treatment to medication or psychotherapy in the management of anxiety. A recent review suggested that effect sizes of exercise interventions were in general better documented for depression than for anxiety disorders. Nonetheless, available evidence showed a positive trend for the benefits of exercise training on reduction of symptoms in people suffering from anxiety and those with chronic disease (Herring et al., 2007). The relevant findings have to be interpreted with caution as the sample sizes of available randomized controlled trials have been small, and there are methodological limitations that affect their interpretation (Carek et al, 2011; Strohle, 2009). In a Cochrane systematic review of exercise interventions on depressive and anxiety symptoms in children, there was a small effect in favor of exercise intervention. However, the authors also commented that the quality of trials was insufficient for a definite conclusion to be drawn (Larun et al, 2006). On the other hand, in another meta-analysis focusing on randomized controlled trials of exercise on anxiety, the findings supported that exercise intervention was superior to control group (effect size = 0.48) and groups on other anxiety-reducing treatment (effect size = 0.19) (Wipfli et al., 2008).

Physical exercise could become excessive

While physical exercise is considered beneficial for anxiety symptoms in both non-clinical and clinical populations, it is important to recognize potential adverse effects of excessive exercise on anxiety. In certain situations, anxiety could be provoked by strenuous exercise. In physical training of sports, high-intensity exercise may lead to physiological responses simulating anxiety, and in the pursuit of perfection and competition in sports, physical exercise may precipitate or perpetuate the development of anxiety symptoms. It has also been reported that overtraining, mostly but not exclusively in competitive sports, may be associated with mood dysregulation simulating depression (Paluska & Schwenk, 2000; Peluso & Guerra de Andrade, 2005). As advice to people with anxiety sensitivity or anxiety disorders, the intensity of physical exercise should be carefully tailored to minimize induction of distorted cognition that exercise aggravates anxiety.

Why and how physical exercise may calm our nerves?

Different hypotheses to explain the mechanisms by which physical exercise may help to attenuate anxiety symptoms have been developed. Rather than focusing on a single perspective, it would be helpful to adopt an integrated model that offers a unified conceptual framework (Daley 2002; Salmon, 2001).

Psychosocial theories

Cognitive behavioural approach

Anxiety disorders are characterized by the simultaneous presence of psycho-logical symptoms of exaggerated worries and fear, and physiological manifes-tations of muscle tightness, palpitations, sweating, flushing and tremor. The physiological and psychological symptoms interact to cause a vicious cycle of worrying cognition with heightened emotional response, leading to significant distress and functional disturbances.

Physical exercise, particularly aerobic exercise, may lead to re-enactment of some physiological symptoms simulating anxiety attacks. Typical sensations associated with strenuous exercise, such as palpitation, sweating, flushing and shortness of breath, are also symptoms of intense anxiety. The experience encountered during physical exercise, if introduced gradually, will help the body to desensitize the physiological signals. The feelings of better self-control over bodily sensation with physical exercise training would have a gradual positive impact on psychological worries and fear in the anxiety chain, when the physiological symptoms are no longer considered threatening and out of reach.

Distraction

Ruminations of uncontrollable and excessive worries associated with fear are core symptoms of anxiety disorders. It is extremely hard for a person suffering from any anxiety disorder to disengage from the chain of worrying thoughts. Distraction theory suggests that physical exercise provides a means of forced distraction from the disturbing theme of thoughts. During physical exercise, the focus of attention is forced to shift away. This temporary distraction may help the person to re-examine the rationality of one's worries from a new perspective. Despite a possible tendency for anxiety symptoms to re-emerge after exercise sessions end, it is possible that regular and frequent practice will help the mind to develop a strategy that minimizes the ruminations more efficiently (Paluska & Schwenk, 2000).

Social support

The practice of physical exercises, which are conducted in groups and over a sustained period, involves a degree of social interaction and mutual support. It is possible that an important therapeutic factor in anxiety reduction is related to the positive experience gained through exercise practice with friends, such as the mutual support gained in yoga group classes, hiking and jogging which are often done with partners and teammates. It is of interest to consider that social interactions during exercise may be qualitatively distinct from the social support that an anxious person seeks in order to relieve anxiety. In the context of exercise, the focus and goal would be on the pursuit for improvement in practice through teamwork. Psychological support developed through such contexts would not be focusing on the distressing symptoms, and may provide an alternative way of distraction by which an anxious person would gain positive experience.

Self-efficacy

People with anxiety disorders have uncertainty about the future, worries and lack of confidence. Through the practice of regular physical exercise, a person usually gains a more accurate perception of the bodily sensations and has improved physical health. Appreciation of progress with efforts paid in exercising may help to empower oneself to gain confidence and a sense of control. Enhancement of self-efficacy will hopefully help to reduce self-doubts that will have an adverse effect of rationalizing unsound fears in anxiety disorders.

Physiological mechanisms

While psychosocial approaches help to interpret how one's psychology may be influenced through exercise practice, physiological mechanisms relating exercise and anxiety are important in helping us to appreciate how the brain may react to physical exercise and changes in emotion regulation. An animal study has also reported that physical exercise (treadmill running) would ameliorate anxiety-like symptoms, suggesting physiological mechanisms, in addition to psychological explanations, may play important roles in symptom modulation (Fulk et al., 2004). It has been postulated that anxiety is associated with increased activity of the noradrenergic pathway, and reduced activity of the GABA-ergic and serotonergic pathways in the cerebral cortex.

Physical exercise, especially vigorous muscle activity, is associated with release of β-endorphin, a neuropeptide found in neurons of the central and peripheral nervous systems. β-endorphin binds to opioid receptors, possesses stronger analgesic properties and helps to induce a state of calmness and subjective feeling of wellness. Physical exercise is also found to be associated with an increased activity in the major neurotransmitter pathways affecting mood regulation. Release of serotonin is likely to produce mood-regulating effects that help to reduce feelings of anxiety. Apart from aerobic exercise, progressive muscle relaxation and breathing exercise help to regulate the autonomic nervous system. A balance between the sympathetic and vagal tone will help to alleviate physiological manifestations of anxiety with heightened arousal.

Brain-Derived Neurotropic Factor (BDNF) has been recognized for its significance in neuronal cell repair and neurogenesis. It is also implicated in the depression model when patients with depressive disorders are found to have lower BDNF levels and are likely to suffer from more chronic symptoms. BDNF is mostly released through muscle activities. Physical exercise is associated with an increase in BDNF, and the level of BDNF is also correlated with improvement in depressive symptoms. In anxiety disorders, it has been suggested that exposure to stressful situations (risk factors for anxiety) alters the signal transmission pathway of BDNF, which in turn affects synaptic plasticity response, leading to sensitization and vulnerability to anxiety. A recent animal study found that BDNF signalling within the basolateral amygdala may mediate fear-conditioning responses via different biological pathways (Chou et al., 2014)

γ-amino-butyric-acid (GABA) receptors are widely found in the brain, and have been considered to carry important inhibitory functions of different neuro-transmitter pathways. Underactivity of GABA pathways has been implicated in the pathogenesis of anxiety. Physical exercise has been reported to enhance GABA activity, which may modulate stress response and reduce anxiety. In an animal study with rodents, long-term voluntary exercise enhances forebrain GABA synthesis capacity in the forebrain GABA-ergic system that may be implicated in the changes in stress sensitivity and emotionality observed in exercising subjects. Other studies also reported alterations of locus ceruleus gene expression and changes of different neuropeptides associated with physical exercise, which may also enhance calming effects (Hill et al., 2010).

An integrated framework

To explain the complex relationships between different factors relating physical exercise and putative anxiolytic effects, an integrated framework incorporating psychological, physiological and social dimensions is desirable. This will help clinicians gain a dynamic view as to how the brain reacts to stress with anxiety and how physical exercise may modulate the symptom manifestations. Pathological reactions to stresses with prominent anxiety develop as an inter-play of personality predisposition, early life experience and inter-current stresses. Anxiety disorders manifest themselves via an enduring mind-body connection that gives rise to both cognitive biases with excessive worries and autonomic nervous system oversensitivity.

Physical exercise may help to attenuate both physiological and psychological symptoms through desensitization of the bodily discomfort that links with fear and worries. Positive emotional experience gained through enhancement of self–efficacy in physical exercise and social support in group activities may enhance both physiological states and balance of the autonomic nervous system. The favorable psychological states accompanying regular physical exercise may act through neuroplastic responses with alterations of neural networks instrumental to the development of anxiety. (Figure 6.1)

This conceptual framework helps us to appreciate individual characteristics while maintaining a holistic approach in the formulation of a comprehensive care plan, including physical exercise intervention as a standalone or adjuvant inter-vention for different anxiety disorders.

Table 6.3 *Components of Physical Exercise and Putative Benefits on Symptoms of Anxiety*

Components of Physical Exercise	Possible benefits
Aerobic exercise	Re-experience of physiological symptoms of anxiety through strenuous activities with gradual desensitization
	Sense of well-being after workout
	Reduction of muscle tension
	Reduce sense of fatigue
	Improvement in sleep quality
Stretching and progressive muscle relaxation	Reduced restlessness and feeling of being keyed up
	Enhance experience of calmness
	Reduction of muscle tension
	Reduction of physiological symptoms of apprehension
Mind body exercise, coordinated movements, controlled breathing with meditation	Distraction from irrational worries and fear
	Regulation of emotional reactivity
	Alters autonomic responses to stressful stimuli

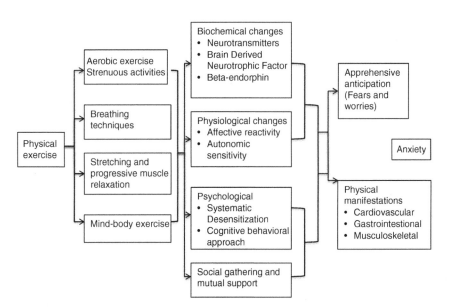

Figure 6.1 An integrated framework linking the modulating effects of physical exercise on anxiety symptoms

Which types of exercise would help?

A common and essential question for clinicians planning to advise on exercise for anxiety is 'Which type(s) of exercise would help?' A broad classification of physical exercise includes stretching and toning, muscle strengthening, aerobic, resistance training, and mind body exercise (Table 6.3).

Aerobic workout

Aerobic exercise improves oxygen consumption and enhances cardiovascular fitness. The physiological changes accompanying aerobic workout may mimic and re-enact physiological symptoms of anxiety, albeit in an artificial and relatively non-threatening situation. This provides a means of exposure and desensitization to symptoms. From another perspective, aerobic exercise may be associated with increased secretion of serotonin and beta-endorphin, resulting in some anxiolytic effects. In a clinical trial on people with social anxiety disorders, eight weeks of either aerobic exercise or mindfulness-based stress reduction was found to exhibit improvements in measures of symptoms and well-being, compared to a non-intervention group observed over the same period (Jozaien et al., 2012). However, in a recent meta-analysis of 7 clinical trials involving 407 subjects, aerobic exercise did not produce significant benefits on anxiety symptoms. Further studies with large sample sizes and more carefully controlled conditions are required to give firm evidence on the use of aerobic exercise as a treatment option for anxiety disorders (Bartley et al., 2013).

Resistance training

This form of exercise focuses on the training of muscles by inducing contraction through resistance. Typical examples include weight lifting, bodybuilding and power training. Resistance training aims to increase muscle, bone and tendon strength, as well as enhancing anaerobic endurance. In a clinical trial (n = 30) comparing 6 weeks of resistance with aerobic exercise training, resistance training appeared to exert a superior effect on reduction of worrying thoughts (Herring et al., 2011).

Stretching and relaxation

A common complaint from people suffering from anxiety disorders is muscle tightness, especially over cervical and shoulder regions. Stretching exercise may reduce aches and pains through either direct analgesic effects or reflex inhibition that induces muscle relaxation. The process of progressive muscle relaxation, accompanied with recognition of ability to relax, would present a cognitive behavioural dimension to train the body to dampen extreme responses. In a meta-analysis of the effects of relaxation training (progressive relaxation, autogenic training, applied relaxation and meditation) on anxiety, 27 studies were examined. Relaxation training showed a medium to large effect size in the treatment of anxiety (Cohen's d was 0.57(95% CI 0.52–0.68) (Manzoni et al., 2008). The effects appeared to be more significant with meditation practice, which may better be categorized under the modality of mind-body exercise.

Mind-body exercise

Mind-body exercise refers to a group of continuous-goal direct movements carried out with special attention to the sequence and flow of postures. The movements are also frequently coordinated with special breathing techniques. Common examples of mind-body exercise include yoga, Tai Chi, meditation. The practice of mind-body exercise is associated with attention and mindfulness meditative practice, which has been reported to exert beneficial effects not only in affective regulation, but also may influence autonomic activities implicated in the generation of anxiety symptoms (Chow & Tsang, 2007; Leung et al., 2014; Wang et al., 2014).

Research reports on yoga and mindful meditation have suggested positive effects in improving psychological symptoms in depression and anxiety, although the studies are still limited by small sample sizes and methodological limitations (Chan et al., 2012; Goyal et al., 2014; Kirkwood et al., 2005; Saeed et al., 2010).

Practical considerations for exercise prescriptions or interventions

While there has been mounting evidence to suggest that physical exercise may exert positive influences on anxiety in both healthy individuals and people suffering from anxiety disorders, special considerations are required for physical exercise to be implemented as a prescription or therapeutic intervention (Meyer & Broocks, 2000). It is important to take a full history into symptomatology, risk factors and personal habits. Most patients may find techniques for breathing and coordinated muscle activities a helpful start to gain confidence in practice, as symptom improvements are more readily experienced. Appropriate advice could on the other hand be tailored to patients who had already adopted intense aerobic practice to optimize the techniques and modalities of practice to benefit anxiety management.

Symptom profile

Although empirical evidence on any specific relationship between symptom profile and exercise type is mostly lacking, the pattern of anxiety symptoms may influence advice on content of exercise intervention. In patients with GAD with prominent muscle tightness and aches, it would be preferable to focus on stretching and progressive muscle relaxation in the beginning of practice. For others who are not very lethargic, but are preoccupied with free-floating anxiety and worries, a more intensive exercise regime demanding constant attention may offer a good means of distraction to help the person to develop self-help skills to distract oneself from the preoccupation. In people suffering from panic disorders and phobia, and with very prominent physiological symptoms, a cognitive-behavioural approach with introduction of exercise practice focusing on systematic desensitization of bodily discomfort, positive reappraisal to correct distorted cognition and interpretation may help to reduce the anticipatory fear of panic symptoms.

Physical health and lifestyles

Enquiries and examination for medical disorders form an integral part of the clinical assessment. Medical conditions that mimic anxiety syndromes should be excluded before the formulation of treatment plans for primary anxiety disorders. It is also important to have a pre-treatment evaluation of cardio-pulmonary status, exercise tolerance and risks of falling, so that safe and tailor-made exercise advice can be offered. A detailed understanding of the lifestyle of a patient will ensure that the exercise prescriptions given fit their personal style and hence will be more likely to be sustainable. In people with pre-existing intensive aerobic exercise habits, further addition of similar exercise is unlikely to offer additional benefits. On the other hand, in people living a very sedentary lifestyle, introduction of strenuous aerobic exercise has to be gradual and non-threatening in this group of subjects with a high propensity for worries and concern.

Logistics of intervention

Physical exercise interventions may not be as standardized or structured as certain forms of psychotherapies. However, it would be helpful to have a framework from which the service could be delivered. There has not been definite evidence as to the optimal frequency and intensity by which physical exercise should be practiced to gain benefits in treating anxiety. The recom-mendation from the American College of Sport Medicine and the American Heart Association for enhancement of health is moderate-intensity exercise for at least 30 minutes 5 times per week, or intensive exercise for a minimum of 20 minutes at least 3 times per week. In the updated guidelines, a mixture of different modalities of exercise has been suggested to offer similar beneficial effects (Haskell et al., 2007). This has been a useful reference for developing exercise advice or interventions for people with anxiety. Regularity of practice is the most important therapeutic factor. As discussed earlier, physiological changes in brain function are associated with anxiolytic effects. A regular and frequent practice would be required to exert the sustainable effect. In an earlier meta-analysis, the results suggested that aerobic exercise had the most robust association with anxiolytic effects for state anxiety. Also, the duration of training and length of sessions (at least over 21 minutes) were important parameters affecting outcome (Petruzzello et al, 1991). There have also been concerns on the duration of each practice session. While no definitive evidence-based answer has yet been available, it is reasonable to assume that a therapeutic session should include adequate time for warm up, core practice, cool down and self-appraisal.

The purpose of physical exercise intervention has primarily been designed to alleviate worries and fear in anxiety. The program should provide a structured regime which was unthreatening with predictable outcomes. It should also help to enhance self-awareness of hypersensitivity to bodily signals and develop ways to cope with the experience. The element of positive affect experience should be encouraged with cognitive distortions corrected through a cognitive behavioural approach. The strategic combination of different types of exercise, such as aerobic training, muscle relaxation, attention training and breathing techniques would not only be user-friendly and efficient, but also synergistic, given the different and possibly complementary mechanisms these modalities of exercise may work to address the heterogeneous etiological factors of anxiety disorders.

Long-term adherence

Anxiety symptoms, either in people with anxiety sensitivity or in the context of disorders, are enduring behavioural patterns. Therapeutic efficacy will only be achieved after physical exercise has been integrated as a lifestyle habit so that a self-generating cycle of physiological and psychological adaptations could be developed (Table 6.4). In consideration of factors that may enhance long-term adherence, it would be important to address the special personal characteristics and optimize the motivation for embarking on exercise practice. The technique of treatment-matching highlights the need to tailor to the motivational stage of the individual. Each person should have his or her own specific exercise barriers and facilitators identified, and programs should be under regular review to enhance self-understanding and appreciation (Martinsen, 2008).

Table 6.4 *Considerations for Physical Exercise Intervention and Long-Term Adherence*

Patient Characteristics	Factors Affecting Adherence
Gender	Competitiveness
	Intensity and Exertion
	Community Popularity
	Social support
Socio-demographic background	Education level
	Financial status
	Occupation
	Previous lifestyles & exercise habits
Symptom profiles	Intensity of apprehensive expectations
	Profiles of physiological symptoms across different body systems
	Physical health status & medical morbidity
Intervention logistics	Frequency
	Intensity
	Content of intervention
	Venue accessibility
Self-appraisal & feedbacks	Positive appraisal of symptom, body sensation and relationships with affective experience

It has been suggested that there are gender differences in the choice of exercise types. Men are more interested in sports with a competitive element, whereas women are more keen on exercise in a social environment. Some evidence has also suggested that women were less likely to engage in conventional physical activity, such as aerobic exercise, but find mind-body exercise therapy acceptable (Leung et al., 2008). Age and physical health status would definitely affect the consideration of exercise patterns. Degree of exertion of any exercise program should be considered from the perspective of previous exercise and lifestyle habits. A person who has been physically active may be introduced to aerobic exercise at an early stage of intervention, whereas a sedentary individual would need gradual adaptation before more strenuous exercise could be introduced.

Feasibility for home practice is a key factor that determines long-term adherence. Advice on physical exercise by trained therapists in the therapy room may be very helpful for demonstrating symptom control. However, follow-up information that guides home practice will be instrumental for generalizing the classroom benefits into everyday life. To enforce positive emotional experience, assistance to self-appraisal or efforts and benefits through the practice adopted from a cognitive-behavioural approach should be considered. People suffering from anxiety disorders are affected by worries and doubts; their cognitive biases should be gradually modified by enhanced self-awareness and improvement in self-control of bodily sensation and affective responses through exercise practice. As such, therapists with a background in cognitive behavioural therapy would therefore be favorable.

Conclusions

There have been a few decades of research on the association between physical exercise and its effects in ameliorating symptoms of anxiety. Repeated meta-analyses have provided some evidence for benefits of exercise intervention, but they do not provide enough information to advise on any standardized form of exercise intervention that fits the needs of all patients suffering from anxiety. The observations on changes of brain activities and associated physiological and biological changes provide support concerning the mechanism by which physical exercise influences affective regulation through alterations in neural activities.

More important considerations have been the applications of such information to advice on physical exercise interventions as a management modality for anxiety symptoms. The complex mind-body symptom dimensions may require considerations about different components of physical exercise to fit the symptoms and personal characteristics in a form that is acceptable and feasible to be built into a behavioural trait enhancing resilience to stresses in life.

References

Barbour KA, Ednefiled TM, Blumenthal JA. 2007. Exercise as a treatment for depression and other psychiatric disorders. *J Card Rehab Prev*, 27: 359–367.

Bartley CA, Hay M, Bloch MH. 2013. Meta-analysis: aerobic exercise for the treatment of anxiety disorders. *Prog Neuropsychopharmacol Biol Psychiatry*, 45: 34–39.

Broman-Fulks JJ, Berman ME, Rabian BA, Webster MJ. 2004. Effects of aerobic exercise on anxiety sensitivity. *Beh Res Therapy* 42: 125–136.

Broman- Fulks JJ, Storey KM. 2008. Evaluation of a brief aerobic exercise intervention for high anxiety sensitivity. *Anxiety, Stress & Coping*, 21: 117–128.

Burbach FR. 1997. The efficacy of physical activity interventions within mental health services: anxiety and depressive disorders. *J Ment Health*, 6: 543–566.

Byrne A, Byrne DG. 1993. The effect of exercise on depression, anxiety and other mood states: A review. *J Psychosomatic Res*, 37: 565–574.

Carek PJ, Laibstain SE, Carek SM. 2011. Exercise for the treatment of depression and anxiety. *Int J Psy in Med*, 41: 15–28.

Chan W, Immink MA, Hillier S. 2012. Yoga and exercise for symptoms of depression and anxiety in people with poststroke disability: a randomized, controlled pilot trial. *Altern Ther health Med*, 18(3): 34–43.

Chou D, Huang CC, Hsu KS. 2014. Brain-derived neurotrophic factor in the amygdala mediates susceptibility to fear conditioning. *Exp Neurol*, 255: 19–29.

Chow YW, Tsang HW. 2007. Biopsychosocial effects of Qigong as a mindful exercise for people with anxiety disorders: a speculative review. *J Altern Complement Med*, 13: 831–839.

Daley AJ. 2002. Exercise therapy and mental health in clinical populations: is exercise therapy a worthwhile intervention? *Adv Psych Treatment*, 8: 262–270.

De Moor MHM, Beem AL, Stubbe JH, Boomsma DI, De Geus EJC. 2006. Regular exercise, anxiety, depression and personality: a population-based study. *Prev Med* 42: 273–279.

De Moor MHM, Boomsma DI, Stubbe JH, Willemsen G, De Geus EJC. 2008. Testing causality in the association between regular exercise and symptoms of anxiety and depression. *Arch Gen Psychiatry*, 65: 897–905.

Farach FJ, Pruitt LD, Jun JJ, Jerud AB, Zoellner LA, Roy-Byrne PP. 2012. Pharmacological treatment of anxiety disorders: current treatments and future directions. *J Anx Disord*, 26: 833–843.

Fulk LJ, Stock HS, Lynn A, Marshall J, Wilson MA, Hand GA. 2004. Chronic physical exercise reduces anxiety-like behavior in rats. *Int J Sports Med*, 25: 78–82.

Goodwin RD. 2003. Association between physical activity and mental disorders among adults in the United States. *Prev Med*, 36: 698–703.

Goyal M, Singh S, Sibinga EM, Gould NF, Rowland-Seymour A, Sharma R, Berger Z, Sleicher D, Maron DD, Shihab HM, Ranasinghe PD, Linn S, Saha S, Bass EB,

Haythornthwaite JA. 2014. Meditation programs for psychological stress and well being: a systematic review and meta-analysis. *JAMA Intern Med*, 174: 357–368.

Haskell WL, Lee IM, Pate RR, Powell KE, Blair SN, Franklin BA, Macera CA, Heath GW, Thompson PD, Bauman A. 2007. Physical activity and public health: updated recommendation for adults from the American College of Sports Medicine and the American Heart Association. *Med Sci Sports Exerc*, 39(8): 1423–1434.

Herring MP, Jacob ML, Suveg C, Dishman RK, O'Connor PJ. 2012. Feasibility of exercise training for the short-term treatment of generalized anxiety disorder: a randomized controlled trial. *Psychother Psychosom*, 81: 21–28.

Herring MP, O'Connor PJ, Dishman RK. 2010. The effect of exercise training on anxiety symptoms among patients: a systematic review. *Arch Intern Med*, 170: 321–331.

Hill LE, Droste SK, Nutt DJ, Linthorst AC, Reul JM. 2010. Voluntary exercise alters GABA(A) receptor subunit and glutamic acid decarboxylase-67 gene expression in the rat forebrain. *J Psychopharmacol*, 24: 745–756.

Jazaieri H, Goldin PR, Werner K, Ziv M, Gross JJ. 2012. A randomized trial of MBSR versus aerobic exercise for social anxiety disorder. *J Clin Psychology*, 68: 715–731.

Kessler RC, Ruscio AM, Shear K, Wittchen HU. 2010. Epidemiology of anxiety disorders. *Current topics in Behavioural Neurosciences*, 2: 21–35.

Kirkwood G, Rampes H, Tuffrey V, Richardson J, Pilkington K. 2005. Yoga for anxiety: a systematic review of the research evidence. *Br J Sports Med*, 39: 884–891.

Kroenke K, Spitzer RL, Williams JB, Monahan PO, Lowe B. 2007. Anxiety disorders in primary care: prevalence, impairment, comorbidity, and detection. *Ann Intern Med*, 146(5): 317–325.

Larun L, Nordheim LV, Ekeland E, Hagen KB, Heian F. 2006. Exercise in prevention and treatment of anxiety and depression among children and young people. Cochrane Database of Systematic Reviews, 3: CD004691. Doi:10.1002/14651858.CD004691.pub2

Lee S, Creed FH, Ma Y-L, Leung CMC. 2014. Somatic symptom burden and health anxiety in the population and their correlates. *Journal of Psychosomatic Research*. Doi:10.1016/j.jpsychores.2014.11.012[published Online First: November 14, 2014]

Leung NT, Lo MM, Lee TM. 2014. Potential therapeutic effects of meditation for treating affective dysregulation. *Evid Based Complement Alternat Med*, 2014: 402718.

Leung YW, Grewal K, Stewart DE, Grace SL. 2008. Gender differences in motivations and perceived effects of Mind-Body Therapy (MBT) practice and views on integrative cardiac rehabilitation among acute coronary syndrome patients: why do women use MBT? *Complement Ther Med*, 16 (6): 311–317. Doi: 10.1016/j.ctim.2008.04.009

Manzoni GM, Pagnini F, Castelnuovo G, Molinari E. 2008. Relaxation training for anxiety: a ten-years systematic review with meta-analysis. *BMC Psychiatry*, 8: 41. Doi: 10.1186/1471-244X-8-41

Martinsen EW. 2008. Physical activity in the prevention and treatment of anxiety and depression. *Nord J Psychiatry*, 62 Suppl 47: 25–29.

Martinsen EW, Hoffart A, Solberg OY. 1989. Aerobic and non-aerobic forms of exercise in the treatment of anxiety disorders. *Stress Medicine*, 5: 115–120.

Meyer T, Broocks A. 2000. Therapeutic impact of exercise on psychiatric diseases: guidelines for exercise testing and prescription. *Sports Med*, 30: 269–279.

Paluska SA, Schwenk TL. 2000. Physical activity and mental health. *Current Concepts. Sports Med*, 29: 167–180.

Peluso MAM, Guerra de Andrade LHS. 2005. Physical activity and mental health: the association between exercise and mood. *Clinics*, 60: 61–70.

Penedo FJ, Dahn JR. 2005. Exercise and well-being: a review of mental and physical health benefits associated with physical activity. *Curr Opin Psychiatry* 18: 189–193.

Petruzzello SJ, Landers DM, Hatfield BD, Kubitz KA, Salazar W. 1991. A meta-analysis on the anxiety reducing effects of acute and chronic exercise: outcomes and mechanisms. *Sports Med*, 11: 143–182.

Salmon P. 2001. Effects of physical exercise on anxiety, depression, and sensitivity to stress: a unifying theory. *Clin Psychol Rev*, 21: 33–61.

Saeed SYA, Antonacci DJ, Bloch RM. 2010. Exercise, yoga and meditation for depressive and anxiety disorders. *Am Fam Physician*, 81: 981–986.

Smits JAJ, Berry AC, Rosenfield D, Powers MB, Behar E, Otto MW. 2008. Reducing anxiety sensitivity with exercise. *Dep Anxiety*, 25: 689–699.

Strohle A. 2009. Physical activity, exercise, depression and anxiety disorders. *J Neural Transm*, 116: 777–784.

Tkachuk GA. Martin GL. 1999. Exercise therapy for patients with psychiatric disorders: research and clinical implications. *Prof Psychol Res Practice*, 30: 275–282.

Wang CW, Chan CH, Ho RT, Chan JS, Ng SM, Chan SL. 2014. Managing stress and anxiety through qigong exercise in healthy adults: a systematic review and meta-analysis of randomized controlled trials. *BMC Complement Altern Med*, 14: 8.

Wipfli BM, Rethorst CD, Landers DM. 2008. The anxiolytic effects of exercise: a meta-analysis of randomized trials and dose-response analysis. *J Sport Exerc Psychol*, 30: 392–410.

7

The Treatment with Exercise Augmentation for Depression (TREAD) study

Chad D. Rethorst, Tracy L. Greer and Madhukar H. Trivedi

Introduction/rationale

Major Depressive Disorder (MDD) is a chronic, recurring disorder resulting in significant burden (Greenberg et al., 2003; Lopez and Murray, 1998; Mathers and Loncar, 2006). Selective serotonin reuptake inhibitors (SSRIs) are the standard of care in antidepressant treatment; however, only 30–35% of patients achieve remission following initial treatment, and approximately one-third of patients remain unremitted following multiple treatment steps (Trivedi et al., 2006a; Trivedi et al., 2006b). Furthermore, those patients who achieve remission may continue to exhibit clinically significant residual symptoms. These residual symptoms result in impairments in functioning and quality of life, and an increased likelihood of relapse (Fava, 1999; Greer et al., 2010; Judd et al., 1994; Judd et al., 1999; Paykel, 1998).

Achieving full remission of depressive symptoms requires additional treatment strategies (Kocsis et al., 2009; Nierenberg et al., 2006; Rush et al., 2006a; Rush et al., 2006b; Thase et al., 2007; Wisniewski et al., 2007). Augmentation is an ideal strategy for partial responders since it allows them to continue using a treatment that has resulted in some benefit (Trivedi, 2009). Exercise may be an effective augmentation strategy for the treatment of non-remitted MDD. Research has demonstrated efficacy of exercise as a monotherapy treatment for MDD (Blumenthal et al., 2007; Dunn et al., 2005; Rethorst et al., 2009) and in combination with other treatments (Blumenthal et al., 1999; Mather et al., 2002). Furthermore, exercise improves common residual symptoms of MDD including sleep disturbances, psychosocial functioning, and cognitive functioning (Galper et al., 2006; Martin et al., 2009). The Treatment with Exercise Augmentation for Depression (TREAD; Rush et al., 1996; Trivedi et al., 2006c; Trivedi et al., 2011) trial was a randomized controlled trial, funded by the National Institute for

Physical Exercise Interventions for Mental Health, ed. Linda C. W. Lam and Michelle Riba. Published by Cambridge University Press. © Cambridge University Press 2016.

Mental Health (1 R01 MH67692-01), aimed to examine the efficacy of exercise as an augmentation strategy for non-remitted MDD.

Study design/methods

Inclusion/exclusion criteria

Inclusion criteria for TREAD were 1) men and women ages 18–70; 2) diagnosis of non-psychotic MDD based on a Structured Clinical Interview for DSM-IV Axis I disorders (SCID); 3) two to six months of treatment with an SSRI, with at least six weeks at an adequate dose (defined as 20mg escitalopram; 40mg citalopram, paroxetine, or fluoxetine; 25mg paroxetine CR; or 150mg sertraline); 4) self-reports of some improvement from SSRI monotherapy, but still experience of residual depressive symptomatology, quantified by an HRSD17 score $\geq$ 14, 5) sedentary (defined as exercise on less than 3 days per week for 20 minutes or less); 6) physically able to exercise; 7) able and willing to provide informed consent.

Exclusion criteria were 1) presence of a medical condition contraindicating exercise, 2) depression due to comorbid psychiatric disorder, 3) current treatment other than SSRI, 4) treatment-resistant MDD (defined as 2 or more treatment failures during current depressive episode), 5) pregnancy or planned pregnancy in the upcoming year.

Screening

Interested subjects were scheduled for Screening Visit #1 at the Mood Disorders Research Program and Clinic at UT Southwestern Medical Center to establish diagnostic and psychiatric eligibility for participation. Subjects who remained eligible following this visit attended Screening Visit #2 at the Cooper Institute to undergo the medical eligibility screening. This visit included a physical evaluation, phlebotomy, anthropometry assessment, and a maximal exercise test.

Baseline assessment/randomization

All in all, 129 individuals met all eligibility criteria, and 126 subjects enrolled in the study (three eligible individuals declined participation). Enrolled subjects then attended a randomization/orientation visit. At this visit, the HRSD-17 is administered to verify eligibility (score $\geq$ 14), and additional baseline assessments were completed. These assessments included the 30-item Inventory of Depressive Symptomatology, Clinician-Rated (IDS-C30) the self-report version of the IDS (IDS-SR30), the Medical Outcomes Study 36-Item Short-Form Health Survey (SF-36), the Social Adjustment Scale Self-Report (SAS-SR), and the Quality of Life Enjoyment and Satisfaction Questionnaire (Q-LES-Q). The depressive symptom assessments (HRSD-17, IDS-C30, IDS-SR30) were administered weekly, while the other assessments were administered at baseline and weeks 6 and 12. Outcome measures were collected prior to the first exercise session of the week, and all assessments were collected by raters who remained blinded to treatment allocation throughout the study. Following completion of baseline assessments, subjects were randomized to one of the two doses of aerobic exercise groups in the TREAD study.

Intervention

The two doses of exercise prescribed in TREAD require total weekly energy expenditures (kcal/kg/week [KKW]) of either a public health dose (PHD) of 16 KKW or a low dose (LD) of 4 KKW. The 16 KKW dose is equivalent to the current physical activity recommendations from the American Heart Association and the American College of Sports Medicine (Haskell et al., 2010) of 150 minutes/week of moderate-intensity physical activity. For participants randomized to 16 KKW, prescribed energy expenditure was 10 KKW the first week, 13 KKW the second week, and 16 KKW in weeks 3–12. The 4 KKW dose was selected, as it represented a sufficient dose of exercise to keep subjects interested and compliant with the protocol while being below the dose believed to be necessary to derive antidepressant benefit (Dunn et al., 2005). The 4 KKW dose is equivalent to approximately 60 minutes/week.

Subjects engaged in their prescribed dose of exercise for 12 weeks through a combination of supervised and home-based exercise sessions. This combination allows for greater scheduling flexibility and minimizes participant burden, ultimately resulting in better adherence rates (Blumenthal et al., 2007; King et al., 1991; King et al., 1995). During the initial supervised exercise sessions, participants were instructed on the proper use of all equipment and on the accurate recording of their exercise session necessary for home-based exercise sessions. Participants completed three supervised sessions during the first week and two supervised sessions during the second week. In the third week and beyond, participants completed one supervised exercise session. Subjects completed the remaining dose for each week during the home-based exercise sessions. Home-based sessions were monitored using a Polar S610i heart rate monitor, and subjects were instructed to submit exercise session data via the study website. Exercise intensity for all sessions were self-selected.

Study results

Of the 126 randomized subjects, 4 subjects (3 higher-dose subjects and 1 lower-dose subject) did not provide post-baseline data and were not evaluable. Therefore, all analyses were conducted on the 122 subjects who completed at least one post-baseline assessment. Demographic and baseline data are presented in Table 7.1. As would be expected, median KKW expenditure during weeks 3–12 was significantly greater in the PHD group than in the LD group (824 kcal vs 290 kcal; $p < .0001$), as were the median minutes of exercise per week (132 minutes

Table 7.1 *Baseline Demographic and Clinical Characteristics*

Variable	PHD group (n = 61)		LD group (n = 61)	
	Mean	SD	Mean	SD
Age (years)	45.6	10.4	48.5	9.4
Female (%)	85.3		78.7	
Race (%)				
White	83.6		88.5	
Black	14.8		8.2	
Hispanic	0.0		1.6	
Other	1.6		1.6	
HRSD17	17.8	3.8	18.1	3.8
IDS-C30	33.3	7.1	34.7	7.8
IDS-SR-30	31.7	8.2	33.1	10.9
Total Insomnia*	3.9	2.3	4.5	1.8
Hypersomnia[#]	0.7	0.9	0.7	0.1

* Sum of 3 insomnia items on the IDS-C: Sleep onset, Mid-Nocturnal, Early Morning (Range 0–9).

[#] Single Hypersomnia item on the IDS-C (Range 0–3).

vs. 60 minutes; $p < .0001$). However, the median adherence rate (defined as percentage of exercise dose completed) was significantly greater in the LD group, 99.4%, than in the PHD group, 63.8% ($p = .0005$)

Primary outcome analysis

The primary study aim was to compare the efficacy of augmenting SSRI treatment with a public health dose of exercise (SSRI + PHD) to a low dose of exercise (SSRI + LD) (Trivedi et al., 2011). The primary outcome was remission of symptoms, defined as an IDS-C30 score of ≤ 12. Exit remission rates were identical (29.5%) in both exercise groups. The change over time in probability of remission was compared between groups using a generalized linear mixed model (GLMM). Results of this analysis indicated that estimated remission rates improved significantly during the study for all participants ($F_{1,1118} = 49.4$, $p < .0001$); however, there was no significant difference between the two exercise groups (group effect: $F_{1,1118} = 1.9$, $p = .17$; group-by-time effect: $F_{1,1118} = 1.6$, $p = .20$).

A covariate-adjusted that included race, sex, QIDS-C16 scores (derived from the IDS-C30 scores), SF-36 mental score, family history of mental illness, recurrent MDD episode status, and the interactions of all these with exercise group also showed significant improvement over time for both groups combined ($F_{1,121} = 39.9$, $p < .0001$), although the group effect showed only a trend toward significance (group effect: $F_{1,134} = 3.2$, $p = .07$; group-by-time effect: $F_{1,119} = 3.8$,

Table 7.2 *Covariate-Adjusted Remission Rates by Sex and Family History of Mental Illness*

Family History	Sex	PHD	LD
Yes	Female	15.5%	43.7%
	Male	62.6%	1.7%
No	Female	39.0%	5.6%
	Male	85.4%	0.1%

$p = .06$). Covariate-adjusted remission rates at week 12 were 28.3% in the PHD group compared to 15.5% in the LD group. This difference in covariate-adjusted remission rates equates to a number needed to treat (NNT) of 7.8 for PHD versus LD, indicating that every 7.8 patients prescribed the PHD of exercise will result in one more case of MDD remission.

Moderators of treatment effect

Analyses were conducted to examine the possible moderator effects of all the covariates (Trivedi et al., 2011). Moderator effects were examined by estimating exercise-group effects within moderator-defined subgroups. Parameter estimates from the adjusted GLMM for all participants were used to compute the initial (group) effect and growth (group-by-visit interaction) effect for each moderator subgroup after adjusting for the other covariates. Results of these analyses identified sex (sex-by-group-by-time interaction, $F_{1,90} = 6.6$, $P = .01$) and family history (family history–by-group-by-time interaction, $F_{1,90} = 5.6$, $P = .02$) as treatment moderators. Post hoc analyses of these significant interaction effects examined the initial and growth effects for the four subgroups: 1) women with no family history, 2) men with no family history, 3) women with a family history of mental illness, and 4) men with a family history. As presented in Table 7.2, remission rates were significantly greater for the PHD group compared to the LD group among both women with no family history of mental illness and in all men regardless of family history of mental illness. Among women with a family history of mental illness, remission rates were numerically greater in the LD group compared to the PHD group, but this difference was not statistically significant.

Secondary outcomes

As mentioned previously, residual deficits in sleep quality and cognitive function are predictive of disease recurrence. Therefore, we conducted secondary analyses to examine the effects of the exercise augmentation on these outcomes.

Sleep

The four sleep-related items on the IDS-C were used to assess self-reported sleep quality. The three insomnia items on the IDS-C (Sleep Onset Insomnia, Mid-Nocturnal Insomnia, Early Morning Insomnia) were summed to calculate an insomnia score and a single-item assessed hypersomnia. A linear mixed model analysis of repeated measures examined the change over time in total insomnia and hypersomnia, respectively. The results of the linear mixed model repeated measures analysis (with the IDS-C time-varying covariate not included) revealed a significant decrease in total insomnia (time effect, $p<0.0001$), while there was no significant change in hypersomnia over the 12 weeks. There were no significant differences between exercise treatment groups on total insomnia score or hypersomnia. These results remained consistent when including the remaining IDS-C items (total IDS-C minus sleep items) as a time-varying covariate to analyze the change in sleep symptoms independent of changes in depressive symptoms (Rethorst et al., 2013a).

Cognition

Of the 94 TREAD participants who consented to participate in the cognition ancillary study, 39 subjects who indicated difficulties with concentration and decision-making on the IDS-C30 item #15 completed pre- and post-intervention testing sessions (20 in the LD group, 19 in the PHD group). Participants completed several tasks from the Cambridge Neuropsychological Test Automated Battery (CANTAB) that represented the following cognitive domains: attention; visual memory; executive function/set-shifting and working memory; and executive function/spatial planning.

Mixed multivariate analysis of variance (MANOVAs) revealed significant group differences in the executive function/set-shifting and working memory domain ($p = 0.0001$). Post hoc analyses revealed significantly fewer errors were made by the PHD group on a spatial working memory task ($p<0.04$), and trends were observed on two additional spatial working memory tasks – another involving reduced errors ($p<0.06$), and the other a strategy score that assesses efficient completion of the task ($p<0.06$). The LD group made significantly more errors on a set-shifting task ($p<0.04$). Significant changes over time were observed across both groups on specific tasks within the attention, visual memory, and executive function / spatial planning domains. The percent correct measure within the visual memory domain was significantly lower after exercise augmentation in the LD group (Greer et al., 2015).

Cognitive performance changes were not correlated with changes in depressive symptom severity, suggesting they were independent of improvements in mood. Thus, both exercise doses resulted in improved cognitive function in tasks within several cognitive domains, with additional benefits observed for high-dose exercisers on spatial working memory tasks. Unexpectedly, decreased performance was observed on certain spatial working memory and visual (pattern recognition) memory tasks in low-dose exercisers, perhaps due to the extended exposure to SSRI that was buffered by high-dose, but not low-dose, exercise augmentation.

Predictors of treatment response

Given the relatively low response and remission rates of current treatments for MDD, there is a need to identify predictors of treatment response. By examining pre-treatment factors that predict treatment outcomes, we can progress towards a personalized medicine approach in which patients are matched to a treatment most likely to elicit a positive treatment response. In pursuit of this goal, we examined clinical and biological factors to determine if we could identify patients who had better treatment response to exercise.

Sleep

We examined sleep (total insomnia and hypersomnia) as predictors of treatment outcomes through linear mixed model analyses of repeated measures (Rethorst et al., 2013a). Results of these analyses revealed a significant two-way baseline hypersomnia x time interaction ($p = 0.0057$) on the IDS-C (with the sleep items excluded) over the 12-week exercise study. This indicates that individuals with higher baseline hypersomnia experienced a greater reduction in depressive symptoms through the 12-week study. This result is of interest, as hypersomnia is a symptom most often associated with atypical depression, which has been associated with poorer treatment outcomes (Stewart et al., 2010). Baseline total insomnia did not significantly predict the treatment outcome over the 12-week exercise intervention. Baseline insomnia has been associated with poorer treatment outcomes for both antidepressant medications (Kupfer et al., 1981) and psychotherapy (Buysse et al., 1992). Our results indicate that exercise is effective in reducing depressive symptoms regardless of baseline sleep disturbances, even in those patients who typically have poorer treatment response.

Post-exercise affect

Studies have demonstrated a positive change in affect in patients with MDD immediately after an acute exercise bout (Bartholomew et al., 2005; Weinstein et al., 2010). However, no study has evaluated post-exercise affect as a predictor of treatment outcome. Therefore, we conducted an analysis to determine if affect following the first exercise session would be predictive of treatment outcomes (Suterwala et al., submitted for publication). Post-session affect was assessed using the Positive and Negative Affect Scale (PANAS) and a composite affect (CA) score was generated by combining the Positive and Negative subscales. A general linear model revealed a significant Group by CA interaction [$F(1,115) = 4.13$, p <.05: $\eta^2 = .035$], indicating that higher CA scores following the initial exercise session were predictive of better treatment outcomes for subjects in the PHD group but not in the LD group. This suggests that assessing affect following an acute bout of exercise may be a clinically useful tool in determining which patients may benefit from exercise augmentation.

Biological markers

As an auxiliary study, participants were asked to provide blood samples at baseline and following study completion; 108 signed additional consent for blood analysis at baseline (105 samples were available); 73 of these completed the study and provided week-12 samples. Serum levels of brain-derived neurotrophic factor were assessed using R&D Human BDNF Quantikine kits (R&D Systems, Minneapolis, MN, USA). Plasma levels of inflammatory cytokines: interleukin-6 (IL-6), IL-1B, and tumor-necrosis factor-alpha (TNF-a) were analyzed in duplicate using a multiplexed chemo-illuminescent ELISA method (MesoScale Discovery, Gaithersburg, MD, USA). Baseline and Week 12 biomarker levels are presented in Table 7.3.

Higher levels of baseline BDNF were associated with a greater decrease in depressive symptoms (p = 0.0046). This effect was further moderated by BMI as indicated by a significant three-way interaction (BDNF by BMI by time). Post hoc analysis of this interaction revealed similar reductions in individuals with low BMI regardless of BDNF level. However, among persons with high BMI, high baseline levels of BDNF were predictive of a greater treatment response (Toups et al., 2011). Similarly, linear mixed model repeated-measures analyses indicated that higher levels of baseline TNF-α were related to a greater decrease in IDS-C

Table 7.3 *Mean Biomarker Levels at Baseline and Post-Intervention*

Group	n	Baseline M (SD)	Week 12 M (SD)	Δ_M M (SD)	p-value
			IL-1β		
All Completers	70	0.10 (0.07)	0.13 (0.27)	0.03 (0.28)	0.38
4 KKW	39	0.10 (0.06)	0.11 (0.06)	0.01 (0.07)	0.77
16 KKW	31	0.09 (0.08)	0.16 (0.41)	0.07 (0.42)	0.2
			IL-6		
All Completers	73	0.89 (0.77)	0.77 (0.52)	−0.12 (0.79)	0.57
4 KKW	40	0.87 (0.75)	0.79 (0.56)	−0.08 (0.79)	0.88
16 KKW	33	0.91 (0.79)	0.74 (0.46)	−0.17 (0.81)	0.52
			TNF-α		
All Completers	72	5.77 (1.74)	5.60 (1.67)	−0.17 (0.97)	0.19
4 KKW	39	6.18 (1.75)	5.86 (1.67)	−0.32 (1.06)	0.14
16 KKW	33	5.28 (1.62)	5.29 (1.64)	0.01 (0.83)	0.91
			BDNF		
All Completers	70	19.1 (6.0)	19.2 (5.8)	0.1 (3.5)	0.86
4 KKW	38	18.6 (6.5)	19.2 (5.7)	0.5 (3.6)	0.44
16 KKW	32	19.7 (5.4)	19.3 (5.9)	−0.4 (3.3)	0.55

Table 7.4 *Spearman Correlation Coefficients between the Change in Biomarkers and Change in Depression Severity (IDS-C)*

Group	n	r_s	p-value
		INF-γ	
All Completers	70	−0.04	0.75
4 KKW	39	−0.19	0.25
16 KKW	31	0.12	0.52
		IL1-β	
All Completers	68	0.24	**0.04**
4 KKW	38	0.20	0.23
16 KKW	30	0.29	0.12
		IL-6	
All Completers	71	0.20	0.09
4 KKW	39	0.23	0.16
16 KKW	32	0.15	0.41
		TNF-α	
All Completers	70	0.05	0.69
4 KKW	38	−0.04	0.83
16 KKW	32	0.09	0.62
		BDNF	
All Completers	68	−0.01	0.89
4 KKW	37	−0.08	0.47
16 KKW	31	0.03	0.79

total scores over the course of the 12-week study. No other baseline cytokine was predictive of treatment outcome in our analysis (Rethorst et al., 2013b).

To further understand the potential role of these biomarkers in the antidepressant effects of exercise augmentation, we examined the correlations between changes in the biomarkers and changes in depressive symptoms (Table 7.4). This analysis revealed a significant positive association between change in IL-1b and change in depressive symptoms. Correlations between change in depression severity and change in other cytokines were not significant, nor was the correlation between changes in depressive symptoms and changes in BDNF.

Future directions

The TREAD study has highlighted the potential utility of exercise augmentation in the treatment of MDD. While benefits were observed with both high and low doses of exercise, the moderating effects of sex and family history suggest that further investigation of other potential moderators is warranted. Furthermore, treatment adherence was greater in the LD exercise group, suggesting the need to develop strategies to enhance adherence in higher doses of exercise.

The effects of exercise on secondary outcomes, including sleep, psychosocial function, and cognitive function, suggest the need to develop additional studies in this area that are specifically designed with these targets as primary outcomes. These symptoms are common residual symptoms of depression that are associated with reduced quality of life and poor overall disease prognosis. A better understanding of the extent to which exercise may serve as a targeted treatment for these symptoms would be of great benefit to the field.

Finally, additional investigation is needed into the potential mechanisms by which exercise may exert a beneficial effect on depressive and related symptoms. The evaluation of biomarkers such as BDNF and cytokines is an important first step in this area, but additional targets include epigenetic and other proteomic markers, as well as evaluation of neurochemical and neurocircuitry changes that may be elucidated via neuroimaging techniques.

References

Bartholomew, J. B., Morrison, D. & Ciccolo, J. T. 2005. Effects of acute exercise on mood and well-being in patients with major depressive disorder. *Med Sci Sports Exerc*, 37, 2032–7.

Blumenthal, J. A., Babyak, M. A., Doraiswamy, P. M., Watkins, L., Hoffman, B. M., Barbour, K. A., Herman, S., Craighead, W. E., Brosse, A. L., Waugh, R., Hinderliter, A. & Sherwood, A. 2007. Exercise and pharmacotherapy in the treatment of major depressive disorder. *Psychosom Med*, 69, 587–96.

Blumenthal, J. A., Babyak, M. A., Moore, K. A., Craighead, W. E., Herman, S., Khatri, P., Waugh, R., Napolitano, M. A., Forman, L. M., Appelbaum, M., Doraiswamy, P. M. & Krishnan, K. R. 1999. Effects of exercise training on older patients with major depression. *Arch Intern Med*, 159, 2349–56.

Buysse, D. J., Kupfer, D. J., Frank, E., Monk, T. H. & Ritenour, A. 1992. Electroencephalographic sleep studies in depressed outpatients treated with interpersonal psychotherapy: II. Longitudinal studies at baseline and recovery. *Psychiatry research*, 42, 27–40.

Dunn, A. L., Trivedi, M. H., Kampert, J. B., Clark, C. G. & Chambliss, H. O. 2005. Exercise treatment for depression: efficacy and dose response. *Am J Prev Med*, 28, 1–8.

Fava, G. A. 1999. Subclinical symptoms in mood disorders: pathophysiological and therapeutic implications. *Psychol Med*, 29, 47–61.

Galper, D. I., Trivedi, M. H., Barlow, C. E., Dunn, A. L. & Kampert, J. B. 2006. Inverse association between physical inactivity and mental health in men and women. *Medicine and Science in Sports and Exercise*, 38, 173–8.

Greenberg, P. E., Kessler, R. C., Birnbaum, H. G., Leong, S. A., Lowe, S. W., Berglund, P. A. & Corey-Lisle, P. K. 2003. The economic burden of depression in the United States: how did it change between 1990 and 2000? *Journal of Clinical Psychiatry*, 64, 1465–75.

Greer, T. L., Grannemann, B. D., Chansard, M., Karim, A. I. & Trivedi, M. H. 2015. Dose-dependent changes in cognitive function with exercise augmentation for major depression: results from the TREAD study. *Eur Neuropsychopharmacol*, 25, 248–56.

Greer, T. L., Kurian, B. T. & Trivedi, M. H. 2010. Defining and measuring functional recovery from depression. *CNS Drugs*, 24, 267–84.

Haskell, W. L., Lee, I.-M. & Pate, R. R. 2007. ACSM / AHA Recommendations. Updated Recommendation for Adults From the American College of Sports Medicine and the American Heart Association. Circulation, 116, 1081–93.

Judd, L. L., Paulus, M. P. & Zeller, P. 1999. The role of residual subthreshold depressive symptoms in early episode relapse in unipolar major depressive disorder. *Arch Gen Psychiatry*, 56, 764–5.

Judd, L. L., Rapaport, M. H., Paulus, M. P. & Brown, J. L. 1994. Subsyndromal symptomatic depression: a new mood disorder? *J Clin Psychiatry*, 55 Suppl, 18–28.

King, A. C., Haskell, W. L., Taylor, C. B., Kraemer, H. C. & Debusk, R. F. 1991. Group- vs home-based exercise training in healthy older men and women: A community-based clinical trial. *JAMA*, 266, 1535–42.

King, A. C., Haskell, W. L., Young, D. R., Oka, R. K. & Stefanick, M. L. 1995. Long-term effects of varying intensities and formats of physical activity on participation rates, fitness, and lipoproteins in men and women aged 50 to 65 years. *Circulation*, 91, 2596–604.

Kocsis, J. H., Gelenberg, A. J., Rothbaum, B. O., Klein, D. N., Trivedi, M. H., Manber, R., Keller, M. B., Leon, A. C., Wisniewski, S. R., Arnow, B. A., Markowitz, J. C., Thase, M. E. & Investigators, R. 2009. Cognitive behavioral analysis system of psychotherapy and brief supportive psychotherapy for augmentation of antidepressant nonresponse in chronic depression: the REVAMP Trial. *Arch Gen Psychiatry*, 66, 1178–88.

Kupfer, D.J., Spiker, D.G., Coble, P.A., Neil, J.F., Ulrich, R., Shaw, D.H. 1981. Sleep and treatment prediction in endogenous depression. *American J Psychiatry*, 138, 429–34.

Lavori, P. W., Miyahara, S. & Rush, A. J. 2007. Acceptability of second-step treatments to depressed outpatients: a STAR*D report. *Am J Psychiatry*, 164, 753–60.

Lopez, A. D. & Murray, C. C. 1998. The global burden of disease, 1990–2020. *Nature Medicine*, 4, 1241–3.

Martin, C. K., Church, T. S., Thompson, A. M., Earnest, C. P. & Blair, S. N. 2009. Exercise dose and quality of life: a randomized controlled trial. *Arch Intern Med*, 169, 269–78.

Mather, A. S., Rodriguez, C., Guthrie, M. F., Mcharg, A. M., Reid, I. C. & Mcmurdo, M. E. 2002. Effects of exercise on depressive symptoms in older adults with poorly responsive depressive disorder: randomised controlled trial. *British Journal of Psychiatry*, 180, 411.

Mathers, C. D. & Loncar, D. 2006. Projections of Global Mortality and Burden of Disease from 2002 to 2030. *PLoS Medicine*, 3, e442.

Nierenberg, A. A., Fava, M., Trivedi, M. H., Wisniewski, S. R., Thase, M. E., Mcgrath, P. J., Alpert, J. E., Warden, D., Luther, J. F., Niederehe, G., Lebowitz, B., Shores-Wilson, K. & Rush, A. J. 2006. A comparison of lithium and T(3) augmentation following two failed medication treatments for depression: a STAR*D report. *Am J Psychiatry*, 163, 1519–30; quiz 1665.

Paykel, E. S. 1998. Remission and residual symptomatology in major depression. *Psychopathology*, 31, 5–14.

Rethorst, C. D., Sunderajan, P., Greer, T. L., Grannemann, B. D., Nakonezny, P. A., Carmody, T. J. & Trivedi, M. H. 2013a. Does exercise improve self-reported sleep quality in non-remitted major depressive disorder? *Psychological Medicine*, 43, 699–709.

Rethorst, C. D., Toups, M. S., Greer, T. L., Nakonezny, P. A., Carmody, T. J., Grannemann, B. D., Huebinger, R. M., Barber, R. C. & Trivedi, M. H. 2013b. Pro-inflammatory cytokines as predictors of antidepressant effects of exercise in major depressive disorder. *Mol Psychiatry*, 18, 1119–24.

Rethorst, C. D., Wipfli, B. M. & Landers, D. M. 2009. The antidepressive effects of exercise: a meta-analysis of randomized trials. *Sports Med*, 39, 491–511.

Rush, A., Trivedi, M., Wisniewski, S., Nierenberg, A., Stewart, J., Warden, D., Niederehe, G., Thase, M., Lavori, P. & Lebowitz, B. 2006a. Acute and longer-term outcomes in depressed outpatients requiring one or several treatment steps: a STAR* D report. *American Journal of Psychiatry*, 163, 1905.

Rush, A., Trivedi, M., Wisniewski, S., Stewart, J., Nierenberg, A., Thase, M., Ritz, L., Biggs, M., Warden, D. & Luther, J. 2006b. Bupropion-SR, sertraline, or venlafaxine-XR after failure of SSRIs for depression. *New England Journal of Medicine*, 354, 1231.

Rush, A. J., Gullion, C. M., Basco, M. R., Jarrett, R. B. & Trivedi, M. H. 1996. The Inventory of Depressive Symptomatology (IDS): psychometric properties. *Psychological Medicine*, 26, 477–86.

Stewart, J. W., McGrath, P. J., Fava, M., Wisniewski, S. R., Zisook, S., Cook, I., Nierenberg, A. A., Trivedi, M. H., Balasubramani, G. K., Warden, D., Lesser, I., John Rush, A. 2010. Do atypical features affect outcome in depressed outpatients treated with citalopram? *International Journal of Neuropsychopharmacology / Official Scientific Journal of the Collegium Internationale Neuropsychopharmacologicum (CINP)*, 13, 15–30.

Suterwala, A., Rethorst, C. D., Carmody, T. J., Greer, T. L., Grannemann, B. D., Jha, M. & Trivedi, M. H. In Press. Affect Following the First Exercise Session as a Predictor of Treatment Response in Depression. *Journal of Clinical Psychiatry*.

Thase, M. E., Friedman, E. S., Biggs, M. M., Wisniewski, S. R., Trivedi, M. H., Luther, J. F., Fava, M., Nierenberg, A. A., Mcgrath, P. J., Warden, D., Niederehe, G., Hollon, S. D. & Rush, A. J. 2007. Cognitive therapy versus medication in augmentation and switch strategies as second-step treatments: a STAR*D report. *Am J Psychiatry*, 164, 739–52.

Toups, M. S., Greer, T. L., Kurian, B. T., Grannemann, B. D., Carmody, T. J., Huebinger, R., Rethorst, C. D. & Trivedi, M. H. 2011. Effects of serum Brain Derived Neurotrophic Factor on exercise augmentation treatment of depression. *Journal of Psychiatric Research*, 45, 1301–6.

Trivedi, M. H. 2009. Treating depression to full remission. *J Clin Psychiatry*, 70, e01.

Trivedi, M.H., Fava, M., Wisniewski, S., Thase, M., Quitkin, F., Warden, D., Ritz, L., Nierenberg, A., Lebowitz, B. & Biggs, M. 2006a. Medication augmentation after the failure of SSRIs for depression. *New England Journal of Medicine*, 354, 1243.

Trivedi, M. H., Greer, T. L., Church, T. S., Carmody, T. J., Grannemann, B. D., Galper, D. I., Dunn, A. L., Earnest, C. P., Sunderajan, P., Henley, S. S. & Blair, S. N. 2011. Exercise as an augmentation treatment for nonremitted major depressive disorder: a randomized, parallel dose comparison. *J Clin Psychiatry*, 72, 677–84.

Trivedi, M. H., Greer, T. L., Grannemann, B. D., Church, T. S., Galper, D. I., Sunderajan, P., Wisniewski, S. R., Chambliss, H. O., Jordan, A. N. & Finley, C. 2006c. TREAD: TReatment with Exercise Augmentation for Depression: study rationale and design. *Clinical Trials*, 3, 291.

Trivedi, M.H., Rush, A., Wisniewski, S., Nierenberg, A., Warden, D., Ritz, L., Norquist, G., Howland, R., Lebowitz, B. & Mcgrath, P. 2006b. Evaluation of outcomes with citalopram for depression using measurement-based care in STAR* D: implications for clinical practice. *American Journal of Psychiatry*, 163, 28.

Weinstein, A. A., Deuster, P. A., Francis, J. L., Beadling, C. & Kop, W. J. 2010. The role of depression in short-term mood and fatigue responses to acute exercise. *Int J Behav Med*, 17, 51–7.

Wisniewski, S. R., Fava, M., Trivedi, M. H., Thase, M. E., Warden, D., Niederehe, G., Friedman, E. S., Biggs, M. M., Sackeim, H. A., Shores-Wilson, K., Mcgrath, P. J., Lavori, P. W., Miyahara, S. & Rush, A. J. 2007. Acceptability of second-step treatments to depressed outpatients: a STAR*D report. *Am J Psychiatry*, 164, 753–60.

8

Physical activity interventions for mild and major neurocognitive disorders

Nicola T. Lautenschlager and Kay L. Cox

Introduction

The introduction of the DSM-5 terminologies mild and major neurocognitive disorders has helped to revisit the current approach of diagnosis and management of cognitive impairment and dementia in older people. The new terminology is more inclusive and less stigmatizing. It tries to align itself with other areas of medicine with the aim to identify and describe with underlying causes in mind. In a sense, the area of organic brain syndromes is ahead of other areas of mental disorders as often a step ahead with unravelling underlying causes. In light of these developments, clinicians working with older people with minor and major neurocognitive disorders should also aim to introduce modern medical knowledge into their management plans and learn from rehabilitation medicine. One important component of any rehabilitation plan is physical activity. This chapter aims to give practical advice for clinicians considering whether to include physical activity in their management plans. For current evidence of clinical trials of physical activity with participants with cognitive impairment, some recent reviews all agree that the evidence of the benefits is growing, but still leave many unanswered questions (Chan et al., 2015; Farina et al., 2014; Gates et al., 2013; Lautenschlager, 2013; Lautenschlager et al., 2012; Lautenschlager et al., 2014).

Getting started

Physical activity guidelines

To date, there are no formal international guidelines or recommendations for physical activity for mild or major neurocognitive disorders. General physical

---

Physical Exercise Interventions for Mental Health, ed. Linda C. W. Lam and Michelle Riba. Published by Cambridge University Press. © Cambridge University Press 2016.

activity guidelines for older adults (over 65 years) for good health are very similar in most developed countries with the recommendation being two hours and 30 minutes (150 minutes) of moderate intensity aerobic activity (i.e., brisk walking) per week AND on two or more days per week muscle-strengthening activities that work all major muscle groups (legs, hips, back, abdomen, chest, shoulders, and arms) (Nelson et al., 2007). More recent clinical trials investigating the effects of a physical activity intervention on cognition in participants including those with objective cognitive impairment have utilised the aerobic (Barnes et al., 2013; Cox et al., 2013; Lautenschlager et al., 2008; Van Uffelen et al., 2008, 2009) or the strengthening component of these guidelines (Fiatarone Singh et al., 2014; Nagamatsu et al., 2012) or both (Davis et al., 2013; Williamson et al., 2009). The evidence for a beneficial effect on cognition is apparent for both types of physical activity, although at this stage the case is strongest for aerobic activity with a growing case for resistance training activities and low-intensity activities such as tai chi (Lam et al., 2011). Given the evidence so far and until there is strong evidence to the contrary, it would be prudent to follow the current guidelines when recommending physical activity for older adults with minor and major neurocognitive disorders, but to modify these according to the individual limitations and incorporating strategies that will promote adoption and maintenance of physical activity in the long term.

Motivating change in physical activity behaviour

Even though the evidence is now strong in support of physical activity improving cognitive outcomes in people with some cognitive impairment, the most challenging aspect of this work is in finding ways to encourage individuals to change their behaviour in order to increase their physical activity levels. Health practitioners, in particular general practitioners, have a very important and potent role to play in this behaviour change (Schutzer and Graves 2004). They see the patient in circumstances where they have sought help or have been referred for help, a situation in which one would expect the message about lifestyle change would be most salient. This was demonstrated in a recent Australian qualitative study involving older adults with minor or major neurocognitive disorders, which reported that older adults have a preference for their general practitioner to suggest a physical activity program (Chong et al., 2014).

Selecting a program

In order to advise older adults with minor or major neurocognitive disorders on how to increase their physical activity level, the practitioner should consider the needs of the individual, their health and medical conditions, including falls history, their level of physical fitness, what the individual wants and expects from the physical activity program, their goals, their personal financial circumstances, their living environment, their physical skill level, their currently performed physical activities, their preferences regarding type of physical activities, their past physical activity history, their perceived barriers to physical activity and their support network. The basis for an individualised program should incorporate the existing guidelines but should be modified to meet the person's individual needs. People with cognitive impairment also face additional challenges, such as increased risk of falls; difficulties with orientation and sense of direction; concentration and planning skills may be reduced, which may limit the choice of suitable programs. For example, an unsupervised walking program may not be appropriate for someone who is at risk of falling and has reduced orientation, or a new sports game skill or dance movement may need to be simplified to adjust for reduced abilities to concentrate or memorise complex movement patterns. The program should start off with simple components with an uncomplicated plan and be progressive in building up to moderate intensity with including repetition. For example, the least complicated program meeting the aerobic physical activity guidelines would be a walking program 3 times per week starting at 15 minutes of slow walking in week 1 and increasing by 5 minutes each week for 8 weeks until the 150 minutes in a week are met. As the subjects increase the time for the walks in each week, and as they become more accustomed to the walking, they gradually increase their walking speed, which is increasing the intensity.

Home-based versus centre-based physical activity

The majority of physical activity intervention clinical trials reviewed here have been supervised and centre-based groups (Gates et al., 2013) with few home-based or unsupervised programs (Lautenschlager et al., 2008). In the clinical trial setting, supervised and centre-based group programs have the advantage of being able to more rigorously administer the protocol, supervise the progress of the individual, give feedback with teaching new skills and to measure the adherence to the program. In the community setting, centre-based programs may, however, have disadvantages, such as offering reduced flexibility for times to participate, have a program fee, or have transport costs or accessibility restrictions for the individual and so on. It has also been suggested that groups should have no more than ten participants, as larger groups could be overwhelming for people with cognitive impairment (Etnier et al., 1997). A supervised personal training setting may overcome this disadvantage and have a further advantage of enhancing adherence to the physical activity program intensity to maximize the physiological effect.

Home-based approaches have demonstrated good adherence comparable to centre-based studies (Cox et al., 2013). The home-based approach has several advantages, such as enabling the person to partake in their activity at a time that suits them, minimal if any transport costs, flexibility of timing and number of sessions per week.

For programs to have optimal benefits to participants with cognitive impairment, home-based and group-based types of programs could be combined with schedules that are more adaptable to the changing needs with different severity levels of cognitive impairment. For example, individuals with mild neurocognitive disorder may be very capable, initially, of following a walking program in and about their neighbourhood without supervision, but if they should start becoming disorientated or experience problems with attention and concentration, then for their safety a supervised walking group or centre-based program may become more appropriate.

What type of activity?

There have been a variety of types of physical activities used in clinical trials with mild and major neurocognitive disorders. Walking, which has been shown to improve cognition (Lautenschlager et al., 2008), has several advantages over other forms of physical activity. It does not require a high level of skill, nor does it have the challenge of having to learn a new skill. It is low cost, it is accessible to most people and can be initiated even with low levels of fitness. Walking programs are a good starting point for individuals who have been inactive and are taking up physical activity for the first time or after a period of low activity or a sedentary lifestyle. Resistance training has been shown to improve executive function (Nagamatsu et al., 2012), and these programs are becoming more available and accessible in the community and are increasing in popularity with older adults. Resistance training is important for maintaining strength and can have benefits for health, including bone density, risk of fractures and falls. The components of fitness important for health in old age include cardiovascular fitness (often referred to as aerobic fitness), muscle strength, muscle endurance, flexibility, agility (mobility), balance and co-ordination. Most physical activity group routines will improve most if not all of these components, but some will emphasize certain areas; for example, resistance training will develop mainly muscle strength, while walking will primarily develop endurance or aerobic fitness. Most centres and gyms offer circuit weight training. Circuit weight training that includes aerobic activities may provide the benefits of strength training and aerobic (endurance) fitness. Table 8.1 provides a list of popular physical activities that older adults may engage in and lists the fitness components they develop and some advantages and disadvantages for individuals with cognitive impairment.

It is important for the practitioner to know what components of fitness need to be developed, so that the program can be tailored to individuals to ensure they get the most out of their program.

The differential effect of various types of physical activity on cognition for people with mild or major neurocognitive disorder has not been widely investigated and is largely unknown. To date, most intervention trials have utilised a range of activities usually categorised as aerobic (for example, walking and cycling) or resistance training. Physical activities that involve the additional use of cognitive skills and or social skills but often are not so physically intense, such as Tai Chi (mind-body activity) or dance, have shown promising results, even though the literature is not consistent. Results from a recent meta-analysis of Tai Chi programs in participants with mild cognitive impairment (4 studies) supported small to moderate improvements on global cognitive function but concluded that the evidence so far does not support a positive effect on other

Table 8.1 *Examples of Moderate-Intensity Physical Activities Used by Older Adults with Cognitive Impairment.*

Physical Activity	Components of fitness potentially developed	Considerations
Walking	aerobic fitness, muscle strength; muscle endurance, balance and co-ordination; agility and mobility	Walking is a very versatile and widely accepted starting activity for most older adults. However, if orientation and balance are impaired, this should be supervised or accompanied and preferably implemented in a controlled environment such as a centre or safe location.
Resistance training	muscle strength; muscle endurance, balance and co-ordination	Supervised programs are preferred, so that correct technique is used. Cost of sessions and transport may limit access.
Circuit weight training	muscle strength; muscle endurance; aerobic fitness, balance and co-ordination; agility and mobility	These can be implemented with basic equipment in the home, but correct technique is important for safety; as a result usually implemented in a centre-based program.
Aquarobics	aerobic fitness muscle strength; muscle endurance, balance and co-ordination; agility and mobility; flexibility	Water safety is important and hence ability to follow instructions essential. Cost and access may limit participation.
Swimming	aerobic fitness, muscle strength; muscle endurance; and co-ordination; agility and mobility	Basic swimming skills are needed, although swimming skills can be learned. Water safety is important and hence ability to follow instructions essential. Cost and access may limit participation. Swimming should never be done alone.
Movement to music	aerobic fitness, balance and co-ordination; agility and mobility; flexibility	Video programs in the home can be used, but the social aspects are usually what are attractive about these programs. Complex routines may be difficult for people with impaired memory and balance.
Tai Chi	aerobic fitness, agility, mobility, flexibility; balance and co-ordination has movement patterns, attention tasks and multitasking	This can be done individually once the skills are learnt or in a group setting. The group-based setting is an attraction
Golf	aerobic fitness, balance and co-ordination; agility and mobility; flexibility	Usually done in small groups, cognitive tasks such as game strategy and scoring may become challenging if impairment is increased. Access and cost may be a factor depending on financial means.
Tennis	aerobic fitness, muscle, strength; muscle endurance; balance and co-ordination; agility and mobility	At least one other person is needed for participation. Access and cost may be a factor depending on financial means. Cognitive tasks such as game strategy and scoring may become challenging if impairment is increased.

Table 8.1 (*cont.*)

Physical Activity	Components of fitness potentially developed	Considerations
Cycling	aerobic fitness, muscle strength; muscle endurance; balance and co-ordination; agility and mobility	If implemented as on-road cycling, all safety measures and road rules need to be adhered to. Stationary cycling is a better option for the more cognitively impaired person. Bike purchase and maintenance may be a limiting factor.
Games and team sports	aerobic fitness, muscle strength; muscle endurance; balance and co-ordination, agility and mobility	Body contact sports should be avoided to minimise risk of injury. If any of the physical capacities are impaired, this may also influence the individual's ability to respond to the demands of the game, affect the team's performance and ultimately team membership. Performance needs to be monitored carefully in this situation.

cognitive domains (Wayne et al., 2014). Tai Chi, particularly in a group setting, may be attractive for participants wanting social interaction in a supportive physical environment. Whilst walking programs tend to be utilised more frequently because of the advantages previously highlighted other types of activities that may be considered are outlined below.

Dance
Dance and movement therapy that includes music as well as body movement which could be sequenced or free form, also providing a social context, may potentially tap into multiple mechanisms for supporting cognition. There has, however, been limited research in this area in cognitively impaired individuals. A study in nursing home patients with Alzheimer's Disease reported improvement in expressive language abilities on the Mini Mental State Examination Test (MMSE) after four months of weekly sessions but not overall cognition (Harkonen et al., 2008). Others reported a similar result in Alzheimer's Disease patients (Kanamori et al., 2004). An aerobic dance program resulted in improved global cognitive function in older adults with cognitive complaints (Barnes et al., 2013). Even though the evidence for dance or movement to music to improve cognition is still very limited, if people with cognitive impairment are encouraged to be more physically active by the music and rhythm or the social contact involved, then dance movements in its various forms will still be of benefit to the individual. Those who have a dance history should be encouraged to continue for as long as they enjoy the activity. For beginners, the movement patterns should be basic and easy to follow and the instructors well trained in the needs of the participants with cognitive impairment when learning new motor skills. If tasks are too complex or challenging, they can contribute to confusion and frustration, and the individual might lose confidence to continue.

Cycling

Stationary cycling has been used as a component of mixed aerobic physical activity programs in studies involving participants with mild cognitive impairment (Baker et al., 2010). Like bicycling, it is an aerobic physical activity and as such would be expected to have similar effects on cognitive domains as other aerobic activities. If a patient has easy access to a stationary cycle or is able to attend a gym or centre, this is a good option, particularly for those who may not have good walking skills, have joint problems, are overweight or at risk of falling. On-road cycling, however, should be advised only if the person has experience with this form of physical activity and is still competent to ride safely. People with cognitive impairment are at increased risk of delayed or unsafe responses when confronted with a situation that demands a high level of decision-making skills, such as can occur in traffic or when the location is unfamiliar to them.

Water-based physical activity

Swimming and water-based physical activities are predominantly aerobic activities. To date no clinical trial to our knowledge has investigated the effects of water-based activities on cognition. Water-based programs are an attractive option for those who have conditions that limit walking and mobility, such as being overweight or having arthritis. Programs that combine music to the movement may have similar benefits as dance in terms of enjoyment and socialisation. Swimming, for those with swimming skills, is an option, as the motor skills may be habitual, and participation in pool swimming does not require a high level of decision making and the repetitive nature of the activity may be of advantage. Learning new swimming skills may provide a challenge to participants with cognitive impairment, but with trained instructors in a supervised setting the skills can be broken down and taught in an appropriate manner. If high levels of technical skill, decision making and memory are required, such as in competitive swimming, this may not be the appropriate physical activity for participants with cognitive impairment. Similarly, with open water swimming such as ocean or rivers where environmental conditions can change and safety may be an issue, this is not recommended. In all situations, water-based activity should not be done alone.

Games and sports

Games and sporting activities usually require agility, coordination, planning, decision-making, strategic thinking and may therefore potentially enhance the effects of physical activity on cognition. To date, there is little evidence to support this notion although one nursing home study reported handball training improved MMSE scores (Wei and Ji, 2014). Body contact sports and combatant activities such as boxing should be avoided to avoid trauma to the head as well as the risk of other injuries.

What do older adults want in a physical activity program?

As stated, catering to the individual needs of the older person is very important (Schutzer and Graves, 2004). This has been confirmed in qualitative research involving people with cognitive impairment where the most prominent theme was that programs needed to be tailored to the needs and interests of the individual (Chong et al., 2014). For participants with cognitive impairment, specific barriers included 'memory problems' and 'lack of companions', and they preferred programs that were easily accessed and included simple and safe activities. Additionally there might be a gender difference to adherence to physical activity programs with women possibly preferring social type activities and men preferring to exercise alone or in a competitive environment (Cox et al., 2013; Chong et al., 2014).

Assessment of fitness capacities for health practitioners

Before developing or selecting a physical activity program an assessment should be made of the participants' medical conditions and their physical exercise capacity. In terms of the latter, both laboratory and clinic-based assessments can be used to make an assessment of the patients' fitness components; however, in practice valid, reliable and easy to administer tests are the ones most likely to be used. Table 8.2 summarises some tests that could be used by the clinician to do this assessment with minimal space, equipment and specialist expertise needed. The choice of components and tests will vary from practice to practice according to resources and the time available.

Field tests that do not need a laboratory setting and are easy to administer are more likely to be used by health practitioners. Some examples of these are outlined below. The clinician could assess all of the fitness components or select specific components related to a perceived area of impaired performance or to match up the participants' capacity with their nominated physical activity interest. Matching the activity with physical capacity and developing programs to enhance areas of poor performance should help to optimise the chances of successful and enjoyable performance and hence maintenance of physical activity.

Getting started

The promotion of physical activity in older adults has been based on several theories of behaviour change and is a complex area for research. In practice, the approach needs to be uncomplicated for both the instructor or clinician and the participant. For this reason, the following suggestions, whilst based on various behaviour change theories, focus on translation into practice. From a review of best practice for physical activity programs for older adults, the recommendation is for interventions to combine the established principles of behaviour change such as social support, self-efficacy, active choices, health contracts, assurances of safety and positive reinforcement (Cress et al., 2006).

Table 8.2 *Fitness Assessments That Can Be Administered in the Clinical Setting.*

Name of Test	Fitness Component	Considerations
6-minute walk test (Rikli and Jones, 1999)	Aerobic fitness The participants walk around a marked course covering as much distance as they can in 6 minutes.	This test provides a reliable measure of fitness, but it requires a high level of motivation to obtain an adequate assessment. May not be suitable for people with severe and/or multiple medical conditions. Not ideal in limited spaces as walking speed will be impaired.
2-minute walk test (Brooks et al., 2007)	Aerobic fitness Participants walk around a marked course covering as much distance as they can in 2 minutes.	This shorter test is more suited to the less physically able and those with more advanced cognitive impairment, especially if lack of concentration and attention are apparent. If balance is impaired, this test has less risk of potential falls. Requires a good level of motivation to obtain an adequate assessment of fitness. Minimal space required to conduct the test.
Timed chair stand (McCarthy et al., 2004)	Leg strength The participant is seated in a standard chair and stands up and down 5 times as quickly as possible whilst being timed.	Only a standard stable chair and a stop watch are need for this test. Not suitable for very obese patients or those with severe arthritis.
Balance step test (Hill et al., 1996)	Dynamic balance The participant steps one foot on, then off, a 7.5 cm high step as many times as possible in 15 seconds without using hand support.	Minimal equipment (stepping block, stopwatch) is required, but the test needs to be standardised. Assistance may be required if the person is likely to have poor balance to minimise risk of falling.
Timed Up And Go (TUG) (Podsiadlo and Richardson, 1991)	Mobility and agility. Also incorporates leg strength in getting up from the chair, and some versions allow for an assessment of gait. The participant is timed whilst standing up from a standard chair, walking three metres and then returning to sit again in the chair.	Clear instructions need to be given and checked for understanding. The surface of the floor needs to be non-slip, and the surrounds need to be clear of any obstacles.
Back scratch (Rikli and Jones, 1999)	Assesses arm flexibility of the dominant and non- dominant arm. Gives an indication of the need for a stretching and flexibility program.	Requires a tape measure only. Suitable particularly for activities using upper body movements.
Sit and Reach test (Rikli and Jones 1999)	Measures hip flexibility and gives an indication of the need for a stretching and flexibility program.	Requires a measuring box or a simplified version using a wooden metre rule. Requires the participant to sit on the floor, so if mobility is impaired this test may not be suitable as the person may not be able to get down and up from the floor.

Strategies and tools for the uptake and maintenance of physical activity

Assess the stage of physical activity behaviour

A theory often used as the basis of physical activity interventions is the stage of change theory (SOC) (Marcus et al.,1992), which is based on the premise that there are five stages of physical activity behaviour: 1) Pre-contemplation (not intending to change); 2) Contemplation (thinking about changing); 3) Preparation (making small changes); 4) Action (taking up the new behaviour); and 5) Maintenance (sustaining the behaviour for more than six months). In the first three stages, the processes that are used to promote the adoption of physical activity in cognitively healthy individuals rely on cognitive processes such as the comprehension of the benefits, increasing knowledge, finding healthy alternatives, making choices, warnings of risk and care about consequences. These are complex processes that patients with cognitive impairment may have difficulty with, so it is recommended that if used these approaches should be tailored to the participant's level of understanding and ability to use them. The less complex tasks of rewarding oneself, exercising with a partner and using a variety of physical activity matched to the person's capabilities should be utilised to maximise the chances of success. These strategies are also used to maintain physical activity in stages four and five. That being said, it is helpful for the practitioner to assess the Stage of Change to determine readiness to change and how much support the participants may need to get started or to restart their physical activity program.

Readiness and confidence to change physical activity

This can be assessed by asking participants, on a scale of 1–10, how important they think it is to become more physically active: '1' being 'not important', and '10' being 'very important'. A low score indicates that that there is likely to be resistance to increasing physical activity levels. Confidence to change can be assessed in a similar manner by asking the participants on a scale of 1–10 how confident they think they are to become more physically active: '1' being 'not confident', and '10' being 'very confident'.

Self-efficacy for physical activity

Physical activity self-efficacy is one's belief that one is able to perform some physical task (Bandura, 1997), for example, to complete a physical activity program such as walking. The self-efficacy may be ask-specific: for example, walking for 30 minutes 5 times per week or barrier-specific, such as being able to continue being active when barriers are present such as when the weather is inclement, when tired or when on holiday. Employing activities that encourage self-efficacy is important to sustain an active lifestyle. Increases in self-efficacy have been demonstrated with a home-based physical activity program in participants with subjective memory complaints and mild cognitive impairment (Cox et al., 2013). The instructor or clinician can support the participants' self-efficacy by helping them to select appropriate activities, setting goals, giving feedback on their physical health and physical activity progress and encouragement. The latter is an important source of social support.

Social support for physical activity

Social support for physical activity can come from family and friends or significant others, such as the instructor or clinician or other participants in a program. It is important for the participant to have a strong social support network. Some activities, particularly centre-based programs or clubs, are a very good option for encouraging positive social support. In the case of older adults and for those who may have health problems, the influence of family and friends can often be negative: for example, by telling the participants that they should 'take it easy' or that they shouldn't be doing a particular activity. Not only the participant, but also family and friends may need information and education on what are safe and appropriate activities. A clinician's involvement and support are often very helpful for the participant to deal with this.

Goal setting for physical activity

Goal setting is an important skill for the development of self-efficacy and continued physical activity. Goal-setting has been demonstrated to be effective with Alzheimer's Disease patients in cognitive rehabilitation (Clare et al., 2011). Participants should be advised on setting SMART Goals: Specific, Measurable, Achievable, Realistic and Timely. Goals should be reviewed on a regular basis with feedback and positive reinforcement such as praise. Clinicians are in an excellent position to give feedback on health-related physical activity and fitness goals if assessments are made on a regular basis with achievement of goals enhancing self-efficacy. They are also in a position to encourage enjoyable physical activities that have some graded challenge so that the participant is able to develop intrinsic reasons for continuing physical activity (Hardy and Rejeski, 1989).

Education and motor skill development

Educating participants on their physical and cognitive health and advising them on how to seek help to develop their physical activity skills helps to promote self-efficacy and to maintain independence. Developing and mastering skills, and completion of tasks are important strategies for building self-efficacy. Encouraging participants to improve their skills or to learn a new physical skill should also be accompanied by advice to seek out trained instructors, particularly those who have experience working with older adults.

Self-regulation of physical activity

Self-regulation and self-management interventions have been shown to be well received in cognitively healthy adults to promote physical activity, as they are individually tailored to needs, do not require any special equipment and are potentially applicable in a community setting (Bandura, 2005). Self-monitoring, goal setting and feedback and social support form the basis of such programs. Self-monitoring of physical activity with various devices such as pedometers or electronic devices such as the 'Fitbit' are rapidly gaining in popularity. They provide a readily available means, at least in the short term, of facilitating a change in physical activity behaviour for people with cognitive impairment, provided supervision is available to read the devices accurately and interpret the feedback information.

Adherence to physical activity programs

Reported retention rates to physical activity programs involving participants with cognitive impairment range from 92% (Fiatarone Singh et al., 2014), 85% (Cox et al., 2013) to 79% (Barnes et al., 2013) after six months duration and are similar to programs in cognitively healthy participants. Reasons for drop-out include participant or family illness, time commitments or personal reasons (Barnes et al., 2013; Cox et al., 2013; Fiatarone Singh et al., 2014). Adverse events possibly related to physical activity programs have been 6–7% (Barnes et al. 2013; Fiatarone Singh et al., 2014) illustrating that these programs are safe for participants with cognitive impairment. Similarly, programs have demonstrated good adherence to physical activity with 73% (Cox et al., 2013), which again is similar to cognitively healthy participants (Van der Bij et al., 2002).

Barriers to participation include costs, lack of transport, perceived lack of friendly environment, access to programs at suitable times and locations (Tak et al., 2012) and no one to be active with. In the latter case, group-based activities may be promoted and participants encouraged to find an exercise partner or mentor to assist with social support and enhance enjoyment. Health practitioners have an active role to play in helping their patients to manage or overcome these potential barriers to participation.

Steps for practitioners in promoting physical activity

The role of the health practitioner in promoting physical activity will depend on resources and the training of the instructor or clinician and the focus of the core business of the organisation in which the physical activity program takes place. It is recognised that not all of the steps listed below will be implemented by practitioners, but this list provides an example of the degree of involvement that could be achieved with adequate resources and commitment. Important steps are:
- Assessing current physical activity level: Stage of Change
- Assessing readiness and confidence to change physical activity behaviour
- Assessment of self-efficacy
- Review and management of medical conditions
- Assessment of physical capacity
- Identification of the patient's needs relating to physical activity
- Goal setting: SMART goals for physical activity
- Selecting an appropriate physical activity and setting
- Identify potential barriers
- Identify self-management and monitoring tools
- Provide feedback and positive reinforcement

- Identify potential for social support
- Provide progressive reports on progress

Conclusions

Reflected by the increasing number of clinical trials as well as systematic and non-systematic reviews, physical activity as a recommended healthy behaviour for older adults with cognitive impairment is considered an important emerging topic when considering best-practice management approaches for cognitive impairment. The literature providing information on how to best translate this evidence into clinical practice is much less developed at present. However, despite existing knowledge gaps, the multiple benefits of physical activity justify that community services and clinical settings update their management approaches with the aim of routinely offering participation in physical activity to people with cognitive impairment.

References

Baker LD, Frank LL, Foster-Schubert K, Green PS, Wilkinson CW, McTiernan A, Lymate SR, Fishel MA, Watson GS, Cholerton BA, Duncan GE, Mejta PD, Craft S. 2010. Effects of the aerobic exercise on mild cognitive impairment: a controlled trial. *Arch Neurol*, 67(1): 71–79.

Bandura A. 1997. *Self-efficacy: The exercise of control*. New York: Freeman.

Bandura A. 2005. The primacy of self-regulation in health promotion. *Applied Psychology: An International Review*, 54(2): 245–254.

Barnes. DE, Santos-Modesitt W, Poelke G, Kramer AF, Castro C, Middleton LE, Yaffe K. 2013. The mental activity and eXercise (MAX) Trial: a randomized controlled trial to enhance cognitive function in older adults. *JAMA Intern Med*, 173(9): 797–804.

Brooks D, Davis AM, Naglie G. 2007. The feasibility of six-minute and two-minute walk tests in in-patient geriatric rehabilitation. *Can J Aging*, 26(2): 159–162.

Chan WC, Yeung JWF, Wong CSM, Lam LCW, Chung KF, Luk JKH, Lee JSW, Law ACK. 2015. Efficacy of physical exercise in preventing falls in older adults with cognitive impairment: a systematic review and meta-analysis. *JAMDA*, 16(2):149–154.

Chong T, Doyle C, Cyarto E, Cox K, Ellis K, Ames D, Lautenschlager N. 2014. Physical activity program preferences and perspectives of older adults with and without cognitive impairment. *Asia-Pac Psychiatry* 6: 179–190.

Clare L, Evans A, Parkinson C, Woods R, Linden D. 2011. Goal-setting in cognitive rehabilitation for people with early-stage Alzheimer's disease. *Clinical Gerontologist*, 34: 220–236.

Cox KL, Flicker L, Almeida OP, Xiao J, Greenop KR, Hendriks J, Phillips M, Lautenschlager NT. 2013. The FABS trial: a randomized control trial of the effects of a 6-month physical activity intervention on adherence and long-term physical activity and self-efficacy in older adults with memory complaints. *Preventive Medicine*, 57: 824–830.

Cress ME, Buchner DM, Prohaska T, Rimmer J, Brown M, Macera C, DePietro L, Chodzko-Zajko W. 2006. Best practices for physical activity programs and behavior counseling in older adult populations. *Eur Rev Aging Phys Act*, 3: 34–42.

Davis JC, Bryan S, Marra CA, Sharma D, Chan A, Beattie BL, Graf P, Liu-Ambrose T. 2013. An economic evaluation of resistance training and aerobic training versus balance and toning exercises in older adults with mild cognitive impairment. *PLOS ONE*, 8(5): e63031.

Etnier JL, Salazar W, Landers DM, Petruzzello SJ, Han M, Nowell P. 1997. The influence of physical fitness and exercise upon cognitive functioning: a meta-analysis. *J Sport Exerc Psych*, 19(3): 249–277.

Farina N, Rusted J, Tabet N. 2014. The effect of exercise interventions on cognitive outcome in Alzheimer's disease: a systematic review. *International Psychogeriatrics*, 26(1): 9–18.

Fiatarone Singh MA, Gates N, Saigal N, Wilson GC, Meiklejohn J, Brodaty H, Wen W, Singh N, Baune BT, Suo C, Baker MK, Foroughi N, Wang Y, Sachdev PS, Valenzuela M. 2014. The study of mental and resistance training (SMART) study – Resistant training and/or cognitive training in mild cognitive impairment: A randomized, double-blind, double-sham controlled trial. *Journal of the American Medical Directors Association* 15: 873–880.

Gates N, Fiatarone Singh MA, Sachdev PS, Valenzuela M. 2013. The effect of exercise training on cognitive function in older adults with mild cognitive impairment: a meta-analysis of randomized controlled trials. *Am J Geriatr Psychiatry*, 21: 1086–1097.

Hardy CJ, Rejeski WJ. 1989. Not what, but how one feels: the measurement of affect during exercise. *J Sport Exerc Psych*, 11: 304–317.

Harkonen I, Rantala I, Remes AM, Harkonen B, Viramo R, Winblad I. 2008. Dance/movement therapeutic methods in management of dementia. *Journal of the American Geriatrics Society*, 54(4): 771–772.

Hill K, Bernhardt J, McGann A, et al. 1996. A new test of dynamic standing balance for stroke patients: reliability, validity, and comparison with healthy elderly. *Physiotherapy Canada*, 48: 257–262.

Kanamori M, Kojima E, Nagasawa S, Nakahara D, Ooshiro H, Suzuki M, Watanabe M. 2004. Behavioral and endocrinological evaluation of music therapy for elderly patients with dementia. *Nursing and Health Sciences*, 6: 11–18.

Lam LC, Chau RC, Wong BM, et al. 2011. Interim follow-up of a randomized controlled trial comparing Chinese style mind body (tai chi) and stretching exercises on cognitive function in subjects at risk of progressive cognitive decline. *Int JGeriatr Psychiatry*, 26: 733–740.

Lautenschlager NT. 2013. Physical activity and cognition in older adults with mild cognitive impairment and dementia. *Neurodegen Dis Manage*, 3(3): 211–218.

Lautenschlager NT, Anstey KJ, Kurz AF. 2014. Non-pharmacological strategies to delay decline. *Maturitas*, 79: 170–173.

Lautenschlager NT, Cox K, Cyarto EV. 2012. The influence of exercise on brain ageing and dementia. *Biochimica et Biophysica Acta*, 1822: 474–481.

Lautenschlager NT, Cox KL, Flicker L, Foster JK, Van Bockxmeer F, Xiao J, Greenop KR, Almeida OP. 2008. Effects of physical activity on cognitive function in older adults at risk for Alzheimer Disease. *JAMA*, 300(9): 1027–1037.

Marcus BH, Banspach SW, Lefebvre RC, Rossi JS, Carleton RA, Abrams DB. 1992. Using the stages of change model to increase the adoption of physical activity among community participants. *Am J Health Promotion*, 6: 424–429.

McCarthy EK, Horvat MA, Holtsberg PA, Wisenbaker JM. 2004. Repeated chair stands as a measure of lower limb strength in sexagenarian women. *J Gerontol A Biol Sci Med Sci*, 59(11): 1207–1212.

Nagamatsu LS, Handy TC, Hsu CL, Voss M, Liu-Ambrose T. 2012. Resistance training promotes cognitive and functional brain plasticity in seniors with probable mild cognitive impairment. *Arch Intern Med*, 172(8): 666–668.

Nelson M, Rejeski W, Blair S, Duncan P, Judge J, King A, Macera C, Castaneda-Sceppa C. 2007. Physical and public health in older adults: recommendations from the American College of Sports Medicine and the American Heart Association. *Circulation*, 116: 1094–1105.

Podsiadlo D, Richardson S. 1991. The timed 'up and go': a test of basic functional mobility for frail elderly persons. *JAGS*, 39: 142–148.

Rikli RE, Jones CJ. 1999. Development and validation of a functional fitness test for community-residing older adults. *J Aging and Physical Activity*, 7: 129–161.

Schutzer KA, Graves BS. 2004. Barriers and motivations to exercise in older adults. *Prev Med*, 39: 1056–1061.

Tak ECPM, van Uffelen JGZ, Chin A, Paw MJM, van Mechelen W, Hopman-Rock M. 2012. Adherence to exercise programs and determinants of maintenance in older adults with mild cognitive impairment. *J Aging and Physical Activity*, 20: 32–46.

Van der Bij AK, Laurent MGH, Wensing M. 2002. Effectiveness of physical activity interventions for older adults. *Am J Prev Med*, 22(2): 120–133.

Van Uffelen JGZ, Chinapaw MJM, Van Mechelen W. 2008. Walking or vitamin B for cognition in older adults with mild cognitive impairment? A randomized controlled trial. *Br J Sports Med*, 42: 344–351.

Van Uffelen JGZ, Chinapaw MJM, Hopman-Rock M, van Mechelen W. 2009. Feasibility and effectiveness of a walking program for community-dwelling older adults with mild cognitive impairment. *J Ageing Physical Activity*, 17: 398–415.

Wayne PM, Walsh JN, Taylor-Piliae RE, Wells RE, Papp KV, Donovan NJ, Yeh GY. 2014. Effect of Tai Chi on cognitive performance in older adults: Systematic review and meta-analysis. *J Am Geriatr Soc*, 62: 25–39.

Wei X-H, Ji L-L. 2014. Effect of handball training on cognitive ability in elderly with mild cognitive impairment. *Neuroscience Letters*, 566: 98–101.

Williamson JD, Espeland M, Kritchevsky SB, et al. 2009. Changes in cognitive function in a randomized trial of physical activity: results of the lifestyle interventions and independence for elders pilot study. *J Geront Med Sci*, 64A: 688–694.

9

Yoga-based interventions for the management of psychiatric disorders

Shivarama Varambally and B. N. Gangadhar

Introduction

Psychiatric disorders constitute a significant proportion of the burden on health systems worldwide, the magnitude of which is only expected to increase. Depression, anxiety disorders and psychosis are the most important of these disorders. Other disorders which need attention are alcohol and other drug dependence syndromes, somatoform disorders, psychiatric disorders of childhood and neurocognitive disorders of the elderly.

Selye postulated that any type of life change could act as a stressor, causing physiological arousal and enhanced susceptibility to illness. Stress operates through the autonomic nervous system and endocrine system (Selye, 1956). Brown and co-workers have suggested that stress (life events) can act as a predisposing factor or as a triggering factor, which may bring the onset of illness and perhaps makes it more abrupt (Brown et al., 1973).

Treatments available for psychiatric disorders are generally classified under two broad headings, namely somatic treatments and psychosocial treatments. Somatic treatments include psychotropic drugs (antipsychotics, antidepressants, mood stabilizers, anti-anxiety drugs), electroconvulsive therapy (ECT), transcranial magnetic stimulation (TMS), transcranial direct current stimulation (tDCS) and psychosurgery. Psychodynamic psychotherapy, cognitive behavior therapy (CBT), family therapy, relaxation therapy, and rehabilitation are some of the psychosocial treatments.

The somatic treatments have come a long way in the last few decades, with the 'psychopharmacological revolution' in the 1980s and 1990s providing a significant number of new antipsychotics and antidepressants. However, though these medications have increased the efficacy of treatments, this has not translated into great benefits in terms of reduction in burden or improvement in functioning or

Physical Exercise Interventions for Mental Health, ed. Linda C. W. Lam and Michelle Riba. Published by Cambridge University Press. © Cambridge University Press 2016.

quality of life (Hegarty et al., 1994). Some of these newer psychotropic drugs, especially antipsychotics, also have problematic side effects such as impaired glucose tolerance, increased blood lipid levels and weight gain, to name a few. There is also recent evidence that the 'pipeline' of new medications is beginning to dry up (Abbott, 2010). In summary, current somatic treatments for psychiatric disorders are still suboptimal and have problematic side effects.

Psychosocial treatments are efficacious in different psychiatric conditions. However, these treatments are resource- and time-intensive, making them impractical to treat large populations, especially in resource-poor settings. Complementary and alternative (CAM) treatments have been in great demand among patients with psychiatric disorders, with some estimates showing that up to 56% of patients with depression have used CAM methods with or without conventional allopathic treatment (Kessler et al., 2001).

Among the CAM approaches, yoga is one of the most popular modalities across the world. Yoga, an ancient Indian philosophical method, had its origins in an idealistic monism, the Vedanta philosophy. The original aim of practicing yoga was union of the individual consciousness with the universal one. Sage Patanjali codified the practice of yoga in his Yoga Sutras (Iyengar, 1966) which essentially describe the rationale and the methods to achieve the objective through the practice of yoga. 'Ashtanga yoga' as enunciated by Patanjali has eight limbs or components namely Yama (self-control), Niyama (observances), Asana (assuming certain postures), Pranayama (regulation of breath), Pratyahara (restraint of senses), Dharana (steadying of mind), Dhyana (meditation) and Samadhi (contemplation). According to Patanjali, these 'limbs' should run not sequentially, but in parallel and are complementary to each other.

The potential benefits of yoga, both physical and mental, have led to widespread use of yoga-based practices for various disorders, although purists argue that use of selective elements of yoga without understanding of the philosophical underpinnings or change in lifestyle is not really 'yoga'. Asana, pranayama and meditation are the most common components of yoga used for the purpose of treatment.

Yoga has reported benefits in different physical disorders (Cramer et al., 2013; Cramer et al., 2014; Tyagi and Cohen, 2014; and many more). It has been shown to be effective in stress management and to reduce neurophysiological markers of stress, and may improve cognitive performance (including memory and executive functions), motor functioning and sleep patterns in normal individuals.

Possible mechanisms of actions of yoga in general are as follows:
1. Generalized reduction in both cognitive and somatic arousal.
2. Changes in the hypothalamic pituitary axis and the autonomic nervous system.
3. Reduction in basal cortisol and catecholamine secretion, decrease in sympathetic activity.
4. Increase in parasympathetic tone.
5. Reductions in metabolic rate and oxygen consumption and salutary effects on cognitive activity and cerebral neurophysiology.

Yoga-based interventions for psychiatric disorders

Yoga-based practices have been used for the prevention and management of stress-related mental disorders such as anxiety and depression. Systematic research in this area, however, is fairly recent, with a review in 2005 finding that the evidence was not strong enough to make any specific recommendations as regular treatment for these disorders (Pilkington et al., 2005). In the last few years, there has seen an exponential rise in studies of yoga in psychiatric disorders, with recent reviews for yoga being an efficacious treatment strategy for Major Depression (Ravindran and Da Silva, 2013) and psychosis (Bangalore and Varambally, 2012). Although yoga-based intervention has been used as a sole treatment in some studies, research seems to indicate that a combination of conventional and complementary treatments may provide better outcomes.

Yoga therapy has been evaluated in the following disorders:

- Major depressive disorder and dysthymia
- Psychosis and schizophrenia
- Anxiety and obsessive compulsive disorder
- Alcohol and other drug-dependence syndromes
- Somatoform disorders and insomnia
- Autism and attention deficit hyperactivity disorder
- Neurocognitive disorders of the elderly

Yoga for depressive disorders

Depressive disorder is the most prevalent mental illness. It causes high morbidity and burden, for the sufferers, their families, and society. It also leads to direct and indirect loss of life by deliberate self-harm and alcohol/drug addiction.

Current treatments for depression include antidepressant medications, electroconvulsive therapy (ECT) and cognitive behavioural therapy (CBT). However, these have several limitations as discussed above, including suboptimal response and adverse effects of medication.

Yoga is one of the CAM approaches used extensively for patients suffering from depression. A systematic review (Uebelacker et al., 2010) suggested that yoga may be an alternative to, or a good way to augment current depression treatment strategies. The review also detailed plausible biological, psychological and behavioural mechanisms by which yoga may have an impact on depression. However, the authors cautioned that while results from existing trials were encouraging, they should be viewed as very preliminary because the trials, as a group, suffered from substantial methodological limitations, and that the effect sizes of different comparative trials varied. A detailed review (Da Silva et al., 2009) enumerated nine randomized controlled trials (RCT's), six open trials and one case series in major depression.

A multi-intervention RCT compared yoga monotherapy with ayurvedic medicine and wait-listed controls in elderly patients with MDD and found yoga superior in reducing depressive symptoms. The benefits were sustained up to six months of follow-up (Krishnamurthy and Telles, 2007). Another RCT using Iyengar yoga as monotherapy found that it improved mild depression and anxiety in adolescent patients as compared to wait-list control (Woolery et al., 2004). An open trial of Iyengar yoga, as adjunct to antidepressants, reported improvements in residual depressive symptoms and anxiety (Shapiro et al., 2007). An open trial of hatha yoga in psychiatric inpatients with varying mood disorders, psychotic disorders and personality disorders found that one session of yoga, added to existing medication resulted in significant improvement in depressive and anxiety symptoms (Lavey et al., 2005). An RCT included patients with varying depressive disorders who all received psychoeducation, with one group receiving yoga and meditation, and another group receiving hypnosis, in addition to psychoeducation. Though there was no significant difference among groups in terms of symptom reduction, more patients in the yoga group achieved remission at nine-month follow-up (Butler et al., 2008).

The clinical guidelines released by the Canadian Network for Mood and Anxiety Treatments (CANMAT) for the management of major depressive disorder in adults in 2009 stated that there was reasonable evidence for the use of yoga in MDD (Ravindran et al., 2009). A meta-analysis in 2011 concluded that yoga was effective as an adjunct treatment for depression and anxiety (Cabral et al., 2012), and a systematic review in 2013 concluded that yoga has Level-3 evidence of benefit as an adjunctive treatment for unipolar depression (Ravindran and Da Silva, 2013).

A recent non-randomized trial included 137 outpatients with DSM–IV major depression. Patients received one of the three treatments per their choice: yoga only, drugs only, or both. A validated generic yoga module (Naveen et al., 2013a) was taught over a month (at least 12 sessions) for patients in the yoga groups. Patients were assessed at baseline, after 1 and 3 months on Depression and Clinical Global Impression (Severity) scales: 58 patients completed the study period with all assessments. The results showed that patients in all three arms obtained a reduction in depression scores as well as clinical severity. However, both yoga groups (with or without drugs) were significantly better than the drugs-only group. A higher proportion of patients remitted in the yoga groups compared with the drugs-only group (Gangadhar et al., 2013).

A summary of controlled yoga trials in depression is presented in Table 9.1.

Biological correlates of the effect of yoga in depression

Apart from effects on clinical symptoms, yoga has been shown to 'correct' biological parameters which may be abnormal in depression. Low pretreatment P300 event-related potential (ERP) amplitude was shown to 'normalize' in patients with both MDD and dysthymia (Murthy et al., 1997). In patients with alcohol dependence and depressive symptoms, yoga reduced both depression scores and serum cortisol (Vedamurthachar et al., 2006). In the recent comparative trial (Gangadhar et al., 2013), serum brain-derived neurotrophic factor

Table 9.1 *Summary of Controlled Trials of Yoga in Depression*

Author/ year	Sample	Yoga Technique	Control	Duration of Yoga	Results
Khumar et al., 1993	MDD (n = 50) RCT	Shavasana yoga (n = 25)	No treatment (n = 25)	4 weeks	Yoga significantly superior
Janakiramaiah et al., 2000	DSM IV MDD (n = 45) RCT; 3 groups	SKY (n = 15)	ECT (3/week) and adequate dose of Imipramine (n = 15 each)	4 days/week for 4 weeks	Significant reductions in HDRS and BDI scores in all 3 groups; ECT superior, improvement similar in IMN and SKY groups.
Rohini et al., 2000	DSM-IV MDD (n = 30)	SKY (n = 15)	Partial SKY (without cyclical breathing) (n = 15)	4 weeks	Reduced BDI scores in both groups; no difference between total and partial SKY at 4 weeks Remission: 12 SKY subjects and 7 partial SKY subjects
Woolery et al., 2004	MDD (n = 28) RCT; 2 groups	Iyengar yoga mono-therapy (n = 13)	Wait-list control (n = 15)	5 weeks	Yoga significantly superior in reducing depression
Sharma et al., 2005	DSM IV MDD (n = 30) RCT; 2 groups	Sahaj yoga meditation + antidepressants (n = 15)	Antidepressants (n = 15)	8 weeks	HDRS scores were significantly lower after 8 weeks in group 1 in comparison with group II
Krishnamurthy and Telles, 2007	MDD (n = 69) RCT; 3 groups	Yoga monotherapy (n = 23)	Ayurvedic medicine and wait-list control (n = 23 each)	24 weeks	Yoga significantly superior
Butler et al., 2008	Total n = 46 DSM IV MDD (n = 23) Dysthymia (n = 23) RCT; 3 groups	Meditation + Hatha yoga + psychoeducation (n = 15)	Group therapy with hypnosis+ psychoeducation (n = 15) Psychoeducation alone (n = 16)	8 weekly sessions, 1 four-hour retreat & 1 booster session at 12 weeks.	No difference between groups in HDRS' scores at 6/ 9 months. Meditation + yoga group had higher remission rate (73%) than other 2 groups (62% & 36%) at 9 months.
Gangadhar et al., 2013	DSM IV MDD (n = 137) Non-randomized trial; 3 groups	Yoga module only (n = 23) yoga + medication (n = 36)	Standard antidepressant medi-cation (n = 78)	2 weeks daily + 2 weekly sessions; Booster session in 2nd and 3rd month	58 patients completed All groups obtained reduction in depression scores Both yoga groups significantly better than drugs-only group. Higher proportion of patients remitted in the yoga groups

(BDNF) rose in patients after three months of yoga therapy, and there was a significant positive correlation between fall in Hamilton depression rating scale (HDRS) and rise in serum BDNF levels in the group receiving yoga alone (Naveen et al., 2013b).

Yoga for psychosis

Psychoses, schizophrenia in particular, cause severe morbidity and disability. The lifetime prevalence of psychosis is more than 3% of the general population (Perala et al., 2007). In spite of significant advances in understanding and treatment of psychosis, the prognosis remains difficult in nearly 40–50% of patients (Hegarty et al., 1994). Among the symptom dimensions, the positive symptoms (delusions, hallucinations and formal thought disorder) are easily identifiable and respond well to available treatments. However, the negative symptoms (amotivation, anhedonia, emotional blunting and poor insight) and cognitive deficits are also primary features of psychosis, and in fact may precede the onset of positive symptoms by months or years. These dimensions are more difficult to treat with available treatments (Buckley and Stahl, 2007), and cause more disability. The negative symptoms have also been well correlated with real-life functioning, and have a strong bearing on productivity of the individual. Along with neuro-cognitive deficits, specific deficits in social cognition have been demonstrated in these patients, which significantly influence real-world functioning and prognosis (Hofer et al., 2009; Kee et al., 2003).

Hence, complementary treatment options have emerged as a critical area of research, with various combinations of psychosocial therapies, including yoga. Although yoga-based interventions are effective in a variety of psychiatric disorders, the area of yoga as a therapy for psychosis remained uncharted territory till the early years of the twenty-first century. The possible reasons for this may be that there are some reports that meditative practices may worsen or provoke psychotic symptoms (Walsh and Roche, 1979), along with the perception that patients with psychosis may not be able to understand and follow yoga protocols. In view of these concerns, an important point to be noted in the studies listed below is that the components of all the yoga modules were mainly yogasana and pranayama. Meditative practices have been avoided in view of possible provocation of psychosis, as well as difficulty in verifying the actual practice of the procedure itself.

One of the first studies to use yoga-based practices in patients with psychosis was by Nagendra et al. (2000). This study included institutionalized patients with schizophrenia, who were able learn the yoga under supervision. The yoga module produced some benefits in social and cognitive domains without causing disturbing side effects. A randomized controlled study of a specific yoga-based module for psychosis was published in 2007 (Duraiswamy et al., 2007). This study had 61 consenting outpatients with symptoms of moderate intensity. Subjects were randomly allotted to either the yoga module or a standard set of physical exercises, and were trained for one month (at least 12 hourly sessions) by the same instructors. The patients were advised to continue the practices at home for the next three months. Assessments of the patients' symptomatology was based on the positive and negative syndrome scale for schizophrenia (PANSS) (Kay et al., 1987), and social functioning was evaluated using the Social and Occupational Functioning Scale (SOFS) (Saraswat et al., 2006). The results showed that the scores on negative syndrome and social dysfunction dropped in both groups over the four months, but the patients in the yoga group performed significantly better. However, this study had some limitations; a modest sample size, lack of a non-intervention control group and lack of measures of cognition. Another study from India evaluated a yoga module as a cognitive remediation technique in patients with schizophrenia and bipolar disorder (Bhatia et al., 2012). The results demonstrated the positive effects of the yoga module on several cognitive functions, especially in schizophrenia. A randomized controlled pilot study included 18 institutionalized patients with schizophrenia and allotted them to either 8 weeks of a yoga module which included postures, breathing exercises, and relaxation, or a wait-list group. The results showed significant improvements in both positive and negative symptom scores on the PANSS, as well as quality of life, in the yoga group as compared to the wait-list group (Visceglia and Lewis, 2011).

The findings of the study quoted above (Duraiswamy et al., 2007) were replicated by an RCT by the same group, which included 120 consenting patients stabilized on antipsychotic medications and used the same yoga and physical exercise modules (Varambally et al., 2012). This study which is the largest published RCT of yoga for psychosis till date, had 3 arms: yoga, physical exercise and wait-list. The methodology was fairly similar to the earlier study, with patients receiving 12 supervised sessions or more in the first month. The subjective judgment of learning yogasana well enough to be practiced at home (as assessed by the yoga instructors) was satisfactory in all patients. Family members were encouraged to motivate patients to adhere to the yoga/exercise sessions as regularly as possible in the next three months. The patients were assessed on the PANSS, SOFAS and a standardized tool for social cognition, the Tool for Recognition of Emotions in Neuropsychiatric Disorders (TRENDS) (Behere et al., 2008) by an independent rater. The results of PANSS rating were replicated as in the earlier study, with more patients in the yoga group improving significantly than those in the other two groups, particularly in negative symptoms and socio-occupational functioning. The likelihood of improvement in the yoga group in terms of negative symptoms was about five times greater than the wait-list group and the exercise group on odds ratio analysis. With regard to the scores on TRENDS, the patients in the yoga group had lower scores at baseline, which improved significantly in the yoga group from baseline to the second month as well as to the end of the study. No significant change occurred in either exercise or wait-listed patients (Behere et al., 2011). A pooled analysis of the two RCTs confirmed the effectiveness of yoga for negative symptoms and socio-occupational functioning, with a better effect size (Varambally et al., 2010). On the basis of these studies, the recent NICE guidelines for management of schizophrenia recommended yoga as a complementary intervention, but also emphasized the need for more systematic research in this direction (http://guidance.nice.org.uk/CG178).

Most of the above studies of yoga-based modules as an intervention in patients with schizophrenia were done in chronic patients stabilized on anti-psychotics. It is now well accepted that the duration of illness is an important predictor of prognosis, and interventions delivered earlier in the course of the illness are likely to be more effective in changing the outcome. In this light, a recent trial yoga in the acute phase of inpatient treatment in psychosis (Manjunath et al., 2013), assumes significance. This study was performed using a randomized controlled single blind design, and the same modules as in the above study (Varambally et al., 2012). Consenting in patients with psychosis (n = 88) were included and were randomized into yoga therapy group ($n = 44$) and physical exercise group ($n = 44$). The interventions were provided as early as possible after admission. Sixty patients completed the study period of six weeks. At the end of six weeks, patients in the yoga group had significantly lower mean scores on Clinical Global Impression Severity (CGIS), PANSS and Hamilton Depression Rating Scale (HDRS). Repeated measure analysis of variance detected an advantage for yoga over exercise in reducing the clinical CGIS and HDRS scores. The study concluded that adding yoga intervention to standard pharmacological treatment is feasible and may be beneficial, even in the early and acute stage of psychosis. However, whether these effects of early introduction of yoga translate into measurable improvements in prognosis is something that needs to be investigated.

A summary of controlled trials of yoga in psychosis is provided in Table 9.2.

Biological correlates of the effect of yoga in psychosis

As mentioned above, yoga-based interventions were associated with improvements in psychopathology in patients with psychosis. Changes in oxytocin during the practice of yoga have been evaluated in a recent study which used the same yoga module as in the studies by Duraiswamy and Varambally. This study randomized consenting patients with schizophrenia to receive yoga or remain wait-listed for one month. The patients who participated demonstrated significant benefits in emotional recognition (TRENDS scores) following yoga. Oxytocin levels rose significantly in the yoga group, with no corresponding change in the wait-listed group (Jayaram et al., 2013). Research on the effects of yoga practices on other biological correlates in patients with schizophrenia such as levels of brain derived neurotrophic factor (BDNF), changes in levels of serum cortisol and insulin, p300 amplitude and latency, and neuroimaging studies of brain structure and functioning, as observed in other conditions, may enhance our understanding of the mechanisms of action of yoga in this complex disorder. A review of the research in yoga therapy for schizophrenia (Bangalore and Varambally, 2012) summarizes some of these issues and provides directions for future research in this area.

Table 9.2 *Summary of Controlled Trials of Yoga in Psychosis (All as Adjunct to Medications)*

Author/Year	Sample	Yoga Technique	Control	Duration of Yoga	Results
Nagendra, 2000	Institutionalized patients with chronic schizophrenia (n = 26)	Integrated yoga therapy	Physical exercise	1 year	Both groups improved in anxiety and social avoidance; yoga group also improved in blunted affect, somatic concern and attention
Duraiswamy et al., 2007	Schizophrenia (n = 61)	Yoga module with asana and pranayama (n = 31)	Physical exercise (n = 30)	4 months	Patients in the yoga group significantly better in PANSS scores, functioning, and quality of life
Visceglia and Lewis, 2011	Schizophrenia (n = 18)	Personalized yoga module (n = 10)	Wait-list (n = 8)	8 weeks; twice weekly sessions	Yoga group obtained significantly greater improvements in PANSS scores and perceived quality of life
Bhatia et al., 2012	Schizophrenia (n = 88)	Yoga module with asana and pranayama (n = 65)	Treatment as usual (n = 23)	3 weeks	Yoga group showed greater improvement with regard to measures of attention; changes more prominent among men.
Varambally et al., 2012	Schizophrenia (n = 119) RCT; 3 groups	Yoga module with asana and pranayama (n = 46)	Physical exercise (n = 36) Wait-list (n = 37)	4 months	More patients in yoga group improved in PANSS negative and total scores and functioning
Manjunath et al., 2013	Non-affective psychosis (n = 88)	Yoga module with asana and pranayama (n = 44)	Physical exercise (n = 44)	6 weeks	Patients in the yoga group had (CGIS), PANSS total, and HDRS
Jayaram et al., 2013	Schizophrenia (n = 43)	Yoga module with asana and pranayama (n = 15)	Wait-list (n = 28)	4 weeks	Yoga group significantly improved in functioning and TRENDS scores; increase in plasma oxytocin levels as compared with the wait-list group.

Yoga for anxiety disorders

Anxiety is the commonest symptom in clinical practice, and anxiety disorders are one of the commonest psychiatric disorders. They can be classified under various categories, such as generalized anxiety disorder (GAD), panic disorder, phobic disorder, obsessive compulsive disorder (OCD). Although medications help some of the symptoms in patients with anxiety disorders, most patients have incomplete response to medication alone. Several psychological therapies have demonstrated success in reducing anxiety symptoms, mainly focusing on cognitive-behavioural models and relaxation techniques to manage anxiety.

Yoga-based practices have been demonstrated to cause changes in the neurophysiological markers of stress and anxiety like GSR and stress hormone levels. Yoga has also been tried as a treatment for anxiety disorders. However, systematic research in this area has been minimal, and a systematic review in 2005 (Kirkwood et al., 2005) suggested that there was not enough evidence to definitely conclude that yoga was an effective treatment for anxiety disorders.

Most available studies are in adult populations, but have small sample sizes and effect sizes.

One of the yoga-based techniques with reasonable evidence in patients with anxiety disorders is Mindfulness-Based Stress Reduction (MBSR). An open trial of MBSR by Kabat-Zinn and others significantly improved anxiety and co-morbid depressive symptoms in 20 of 22 patients with GAD or panic disorder, as monotherapy or as an add-on to medication (Kabat-Zinn et al., 1992). The treatment effects were evident at post-intervention and 3 months follow-up. Of note, a 3-year follow-up of this cohort (18 of the original 22 patients) reported that the gains were maintained after 3 years on the Hamilton and Beck anxiety scales as well as on the respective depression scales. The majority of subjects were reported to be compliant with the meditation practice. An RCT of MBSR including 76 patients with panic disorder with or without agoraphobia (PD/AG), social anxiety disorder (SAD) and GAD reported that patients who completed treatment improved significantly on all outcome measures compared to wait-listed controls. The study reported medium to large effect sizes on measures of anxiety, and a large effect size for symptoms of depression, and also that the gains were maintained at six months follow-up (Vollestad et al., 2011). A systematic review and meta-analysis of mindfulness- and acceptance-based interventions (MABIs) for anxiety disorders published in 2012 evaluated 19 studies and reported an overall between-group effect size of 0.83 for anxiety symptoms and 0.72 for depression symptoms in controlled studies. The authors concluded that MABIs are associated with substantial reductions in symptoms of anxiety and co-morbid depressive symptoms, but that more research is needed to determine their efficacy compared to current treatments, and to clarify the contribution of processes of mindfulness and acceptance to the outcome (Vollestad et al., 2012).

Yoga for substance use disorders

Psychotropic substance abuse contributes heavily to healthcare burden, accidents, and increased prevalence of other mental illnesses and suicide. Co-morbid substance use is extremely common in patients who present with various psychiatric illnesses. Multi-modal programs including pharmacological, behavioural and psychosocial components are standard managements of substance dependence. Yoga practices also have been used as a part of such programs. An early study by Shaffer (Shaffer et al., 1997) found hatha yoga comparable to conventional methadone treatment with traditional group psychotherapy and in 61 randomly assigned clients on a variety of outcome measures.

A study from Amritsar, India, tested a 90-day residential group pilot treatment program for substance abuse that incorporated a comprehensive array of yoga, meditation, spiritual and mind-body techniques (Khalsa et al., 2008). Results showed improvements on a number of psychological self-report questionnaires including the Behavior and Symptom Identification Scale and the Quality of Recovery Index. A recent study which included 18 patients with alcohol dependence evaluated the feasibility and efficacy of a 10-week yoga package as an adjunct therapy in a treatment program versus treatment as usual. The authors reported that the yoga-based intervention was a feasible and well accepted adjunct treatment, but did not produce any significant effects in terms of reduction in alcohol consumption (Hallgren et al., 2014).

In summary, current findings show support for yoga and mindfulness as potential complementary therapies for management of addictive behaviours. However, more systematic research is needed to understand and match types of interventions to types of addiction, patients and settings. A recent narrative review summarizes the philosophical origins, current evidence and the future prospects of yoga and mindfulness in this important clinical area (Khanna and Greeson, 2013).

Yoga for somatoform disorders

Yoga has been used as a therapy for several pain syndromes, notably with good evidence for short-term and long-term reductions in pain efficacy for low back pain (Cramer et al., 2013). There is also promising preliminary data for migraine (John et al., 2007, Kisan et al., 2014) and fibromyalgia (Langhorst et al., 2013, Mist et al., 2013). A randomized study using yoga nidra (a form of yoga emphasizing on deep relaxation techniques) as a treatment in patients of menstrual disorders with somatoform symptoms included 150 women with menstrual disorders. They were randomized to yoga nidra intervention with medication or only medication. Results showed significant improvement in pain symptoms, gastrointestinal symptoms, cardiovascular symptoms, and urogenital symptoms after six months of yoga therapy compared to control group (Rani et al., 2011). A recent open trial at a tertiary psychiatric centre in India evaluated an integrated yoga therapy module in 64 patients with somatoform pain disorder. Yoga intervention led to a significant reduction in pain scores and improvement in anxiety, sleep and quality of life in patients who completed the study (Sutar, 2014). In view of the paucity of research data and also the demonstration of abnormalities in inflammatory and neuroimmunological pathways in patients with somatoform disorders, further research to confirm these early findings and also the mechanisms of action of yoga in these disorders is definitely needed.

Yoga for insomnia

Sleep disorders, insomnia in particular, is quite prevalent in the general population, and even more so in patients with psychiatric disorders. Insomnia and dependence on hypnotics is a common problem in primary care settings. Various non-pharmacological methods have been tried for insomnia, yoga-based programs being one of them.

In otherwise healthy subjects, there are several reports of improvement of sleep parameters with cyclic meditation (Patra and Telles, 2009), silver yoga exercises in elderly subjects (Chen et al., 2009) and elderly subjects in old-age homes (Hariprasad et al., 2013c). Studies of yoga in subjects with lymphoma (Cohen et al., 2004) and cancer survivors (Mustian et al., 2013) have also demonstrated benefits in sleep quality. Ong and colleagues (Ong et al., 2008) used mindfulness meditation combined with cognitive behavioural therapy in 30 adults with insomnia, and found improvement in several sleep-related measures. A study in 20 subjects with chronic insomnia using a yoga-based module reported improvements in a broad range of sleep parameters (Khalsa, 2004). There have been some preliminary demonstrations but only limited clinical evidence of the benefits of yoga and meditation-based interventions for insomnia. Further research support is needed to replicate the efficacy of yoga as a therapeutic agent in insomnia and other sleep disorders.

Yoga for psychiatric disorders of childhood

Yoga has been explored as a treatment option in children with anxiety spectrum disorders, depression and autism, but most of these are case reports or case series, with minimal evidence in terms of methodologically sound studies (Birdee et al., 2009). A study at a tertiary care, medical school teaching hospital included 24 children aged 3–16 years with a diagnosis of an autism spectrum disorder (ASD). An eight-week multimodal yoga, dance and music therapy program based on the relaxation response (RR) was developed and evaluated, with outcome measured by The Behavioral Assessment System for Children, Second Edition (BASC-2), and the Aberrant Behavioral Checklist (ABC). The study found positive changes on the BASC-2, primarily for 5-to-12-year-old children, and on the atypicality scale of the BASC-2, which measures some of the core features of autism.

The psychiatric disorder of childhood for which there is reasonable evidence for the efficacy of yoga-based interventions is attention-deficit/hyperactivity disorder (ADHD). Medications and behavioural interventions have been the mainstay of treatment for ADHD, but the adverse effects of stimulant medications make them unattractive for many clinicians and parents. Yoga and meditative practices have therefore been explored as sole or adjunct interventions for ADHD. An RCT by Jensen and Kenny (Jensen and Kenny, 2004) included boys diagnosed with ADHD and stabilized on medication; they were randomized to either a 20-session yoga group (n = 11) or a control group (cooperative activities; n = 8). The yoga program consisted of respiratory training, postural training, relaxation training, concentration training and a concentrative technique called Trataka. The children in the yoga group obtained significant benefits on five subscales of the Conners' Parents Rating Scales (CPRS). The authors concluded that yoga may have merit as a complementary treatment for ADHD. However, the limitations of this study, including low statistical power and inconsistency of home practices, make it necessary to caution that the results need to be replicated on larger groups with a more intensive supervised practice program. A study from Thailand used a meditation and imagery program in children with ADHD (Hassasiri et al., 2002) and found a significant impact with regard to lowering symptoms. Another study by Haffner and others (Haffner et al., 2006) included 19 children (12 boys and 7 girls) diagnosed with ADHD and used a 2 × 2 cross-over design comparing yoga training (n = 8) versus regular physical exercise (n = 11) over 8 weeks. Eight of the 19 children were also on medication, and 7 received other complementary therapies as well. This study found that yoga training was superior to the physical exercise regimen on test scores on an attention task and parent ratings of ADHD symptoms, with effect sizes in the medium-to-high range (0.60–0.97). Furthermore, the training was particularly effective for children undergoing pharmacotherapy (MPH). However, a study which included 23 boys with ADHD (Moretti-Altuna, 1987) compared meditation training versus drug therapy versus standard therapy control, but did not find statistically significant difference between the meditation therapy group and the drug therapy group in either the teacher rating ADHD scale or the distraction test. A Cochrane review in 2010 (Krisanaprakornkit et al., 2010) concluded that there was insufficient evidence to support the effectiveness of any types of meditation for ADHD.

A recent open-label exploratory study included nine patients with moderate to severe ADHD (8 were on medications) admitted in a child psychiatry ward (Hariprasad et al., 2013a). The participants were taught a specific yoga module by a trained therapist daily during their inpatient stay and assessed at the end of the first, second and third months by an independent rater. An average of eight yoga training sessions given to subjects. There was a significant improvement in the ADHD symptoms at the time of discharge. Two recent studies with pragmatic methodology and good follow-up have provided better evidence for the efficacy of multi-modal programs including yoga in ADHD. The first school-based study by Mehta and colleagues (Mehta et al., 2011) used a six-week multimodal peer-mediated behavioural program that included yoga, for children between 6–11 years of age diagnosed with ADHD. The authors measured performance and behavioural scores using the Vanderbilt scale. The one-hour program (twice-weekly sessions), combining yoga, meditation and play therapy, was taught by trained high school volunteers; 76 school children with ADHD were included. After six weeks of the program, 90.5% of children showed reductions in their performance-impairment score, a measure of academic performance. The researchers followed up 69 of these children with weekly sessions for one year and showed that improvement on the performance-impairment scores for ADHD was sustained through 12 months in 85% of the students. Almost all (92%) of the students also had improvements in their Vanderbilt scores as assessed by parents. The follow-up study results validated the efficacy and cost-effectiveness of the program (Mehta et al., 2013). To summarize, there seems to be evidence to suggest that yoga therapy for ADHD is feasible in both hospital and school settings, and may produce significant reduction in symptoms as a sole therapy, or along with medication and as a part of multimodal intervention programs. More research is needed to examine specific yoga modules in multi-centre RCTs and quantify the effect of the interventions if yoga is to be accepted as a standard therapy in ADHD.

Yoga for neurocognitive disorders in the elderly

There is preliminary evidence detailing the effects of yoga on cognitive parameters in healthy elderly individuals (Hariprasad et al., 2013b) and in subjects with depression (Sharma et al., 2006) and psychosis (Bhatia et al., 2012). There are also preliminary findings to suggest that yoga practices may have observable neurobiological effects on the structure of the brain, specifically areas subserving memory, in the elderly brain (Hariprasad et al., 2013c). However, there are very few studies looking at the efficacy of yoga-based interventions for patients with mild cognitive impairment or early dementia, and the available evidence is inconclusive (Balasubramaniam et al., 2013).

Neurobiological mechanisms underpinning the effects of yoga in psychiatric disorders

The various psychiatric disorders covered in this chapter have varied etiology and pathophysiology, covering a wide gamut of biological pathways and neurobiological abnormalities. How can we explain the effects of yoga-based interventions in these diverse disorders? Current research seems to point to a unifying hypothesis involving correction of impaired neuroplasticity in these disorders. Impaired neuroplastic mechanisms have been postulated in depression (Duman and Monteggia, 2006), schizophrenia (Voineskos et al., 2013), and other psychiatric disorders. Neuroplasticity has been in fact described as the mediator of treatment response in depression (Andrade and Rao, 2011). In this light, there are several lines of evidence that yoga has remedial effects on neuroplastic mechanisms. Studies in healthy populations have shown that yoga and meditative practices have led to increase in cortical thickness (Lazar et al., 2005) and increased volume of grey matter in parts of the brain important for memory and cognition (Luders et al., 2009). Recent evidence indicates that yoga increases levels of neurotransmitters in certain brain regions (Streeter et al., 2007, Streeter et al., 2010). Recent studies also provide early evidence that yoga practices facilitate neuroplasticity in disorders such as depression, and that this is correlated with improvement in symptoms (Naveen et al., 2013b).

Challenges and methodological issues relating to yoga as a therapy in psychiatric disorders

Although there is great interest in yoga-based therapies for physical and mental ailments, challenges exist making it difficult for patients to access such therapies, and for researchers to undertake methodologically sound studies. For example, in the three–arm yoga trial for schizophrenia discussed in the section on schizophrenia (Varambally et al., 2012), close to a thousand patients needed to be screened to recruit 120 patients. An article published in 2012 analyzed the challenges for patients with schizophrenia to access yoga services (Baspure et al., 2012). Even though most patients and caregivers were keen to avail yoga therapy, the most important reasons for refusal were the distance from the centre providing the yoga service and difficulties in coming for regular sessions. This highlights the need for provision of yoga closer to home for patients and making yoga programs more flexible.

There are several methodological challenges in the study of yoga as a therapy in mental illness; some of them are quite unique due to the nature of yoga being inherently different from other interventions in medicine. The main issues are finding appropriate placebo/control procedures, and difficulties with blinding in yoga research. Many different schools of yoga follow different systems of nosology, and some insist that yoga should be looked at as a complete lifestyle and not used piecemeal as therapy. This mandates a need for broad agreement among yoga schools and co-operative research with medical professionals for building evidence. These concerns have been discussed in detail, and future directions for research have been provided in a recent review (Gangadhar and Varambally, 2011). Another recent article analyzed the links between yoga and spirituality, which is an important component that needs to be factored into research in yoga for psychiatric disorders (Varambally and Gangadhar, 2012).

Summary and conclusions: current status and future directions

There is tremendous interest in using and studying yoga-based interventions as a therapeutic modality in various psychiatric disorders. However, much more work needs to be done to provide a good evidence base for efficacy and also to determine understandable mechanisms of action to explain the effects of yoga in these disorders. Also, making yoga easily available and undertaking of co-operative research by medical and yoga professionals are challenges for yoga therapy and research. Current and future research in this area needs to address these issues in order to make a place for yoga as a viable addition to the therapeutic armamentarium in psychiatric disorders.

References

Abbott, A. (2010) Schizophrenia: The drug deadlock. *Nature*, 468, 158–9.

Andrade, C. & Rao, N. S. (2011). How antidepressant drugs act: a primer on neuroplasticity as the eventual mediator of antidepressant efficacy. *Indian J Psychiatry*, 52, 378–86.

Balasubramaniam, M., Telles, S. & Doraiswamy, P. M. (2013). Yoga on our minds: a systematic review of yoga for neuropsychiatric disorders. *Front Psychiatry*, 3, 117.

Bangalore, N. G. & Varambally, S. (2012). Yoga therapy for Schizophrenia. *Int J Yoga*, 5, 85–91.

Baspure, S., Jagannathan, A., Kumar, S., Arsappa, R., Varambally, S., Thirthalli, J., Venkatasubramanian, G., Nagendra, H. R. & Gangadhar, B. N. (2012). Barriers to yoga therapy as an add-on treatment for schizophrenia in India. *International Journal of Yoga*, 5, 70–3.

Behere, R. V., Arasappa, R., Jagannathan, A., Varambally, S., Venkatasubramanian, G., Thirthalli, J., Subbakrishna, D. K., Nagendra, H. R. & Gangadhar, B. N. (2011). Effect of yoga therapy on facial emotion recognition deficits, symptoms and functioning in patients with schizophrenia. *Acta Psychiatr Scand*, 123, 147–53.

Behere, R. V., Raghunandan, V. N. & Venkatasubramanian, G. (2008). Trends: a Tool for Recognition of Emotions in Neuro-psychiatric Disorders. *Ind J Psychol Med*, 30, 32–8.

Bhatia, T., Agarwal, A., Shah, G., Wood, J., Richard, J., Gur, R. E., Gur, R. C., Nimgaonkar, V. L., Mazumdar, S. & Deshpande, S. N. (2012). Adjunctive cognitive remediation for schizophrenia using yoga: an open, non-randomized trial. *Acta Neuropsychiatr*, 24, 91–100.

Birdee, G. S., Yeh, G. Y., Wayne, P. M., Phillips, R. S., Davis, R. B. & Gardiner, P. (2009). Clinical applications of yoga for the pediatric population: a systematic review. *Acad Pediatr*, 9, 212–20 e1-9.

Brown, G. W., Harris, T. O. & Peto, J. (1973). Life events and psychiatric disorders. 2. Nature of causal link. *Psychol Med*, 3, 159–76.

Buckley, P. F. & Stahl, S. M. (2007). Pharmacological treatment of negative symptoms of schizophrenia: therapeutic opportunity or cul-de-sac? *Acta Psychiatr Scand*, 115, 93–100.

Butler, L. D., Waelde, L. C., Hastings, T. A., Chen, X. H., Symons, B., Marshall, J., Kaufman, A., Nagy, T. F., Blasey, C. M., Seibert, E. O. & Spiegel, D. (2008). Meditation with yoga, group therapy with hypnosis, and psychoeducation for long-term depressed mood: a randomized pilot trial. *J Clin Psychol*, 64, 806–20.

Cabral, P., Meyer, H. B. & Ames, D. (2012). Effectiveness of yoga therapy as a complementary treatment for major psychiatric disorders: a meta-analysis. *Prim Care Companion CNS Disord*, 13.

Carter, J. & Byrne, G. (2004). A 2-year study of the use of yoga in a series of pilot studies as an adjunct to ordinary psychiatric treatment in a group of Vietnam War Veterans suffering from post traumatic stress disorder. Retrieved on November 14, 2014 from http://www.therapywithyoga.com/Vivekananda.pdf.

Chen, K. M., Chen, M. H., Chao, H. C., Hung, H. M., Lin, H. S. & Li, C. H. (2009) Sleep quality, depression state, and health status of older adults after silver yoga exercises: cluster randomized trial. *Int J Nurs Stud*, 46, 154–63.

Cohen, L., Warneke, C., Fouladi, R. T., Rodriguez, M. A. & Chaoul-Reich, A. (2004) Psychological adjustment and sleep quality in a randomized trial of the effects of a Tibetan yoga intervention in patients with lymphoma. *Cancer*, 100, 2253–60.

Cramer, H., Lauche, R., Haller, H. & Dobos, G. (2013). A systematic review and meta-analysis of yoga for low back pain. *Clin J Pain*, 29, 450–60.

Cramer, H., Lauche, R., Haller, H., Steckhan, N., Michalsen, A. & Dobos, G. (2014). Effects of yoga on cardiovascular disease risk factors: a systematic review and meta-analysis. *Int J Cardiol*, 173, 170–83.

Da Silva, T. L., Ravindran, L. N. & Ravindran, A. V. (2009). Yoga in the treatment of mood and anxiety disorders: a review. *Asian J Psychiatr*, 2, 6–16.

Duman, R. S. & Monteggia, L. M. (2006). A neurotrophic model for stress-related mood disorders. *Biol Psychiatry*, 59, 1116–27.

Duraiswamy, G., Thirthalli, J., Nagendra, H. R. & Gangadhar, B. N. (2007). Yoga therapy as an add-on treatment in the management of patients with schizophrenia: a randomized controlled trial. *Acta Psychiatr Scand*, 116, 226–32.

Gangadhar, B. N., Naveen, G. H., Rao, M. G., Thirthalli, J. & Varambally, S. (2013). Positive antidepressant effects of generic yoga in depressive out-patients: a comparative study. *Indian J Psychiatry*, 55, S369-73.

Gangadhar, B. N. & Varambally, S. (2011). Yoga as therapy in psychiatric disorders: past, present, and future. *Biofeedback*, 39, 60–3.

Haffner, J., Roos, J., Goldstein, N., Parzer, P. & Resch, F. (2006). The effectiveness of body-oriented methods of therapy in the treatment of attention-deficit hyperactivity disorder (ADHD): results of a controlled pilot study. *Z Kinder Jugendpsychiatr Psychother*, 34, 37–47.

Hallgren, M., Romberg, K., Bakshi, A. S. & Andreasson, S. (2014). Yoga as an adjunct treatment for alcohol dependence: a pilot study. *Complement Ther Med*, 22, 441–5.

Hariprasad, V. R., Arasappa, R., Varambally, S., Srinath, S. & Gangadhar, B. N. (2013a). Feasibility and efficacy of yoga as an add-on intervention in attention deficit-hyperactivity disorder: an exploratory study. *Indian J Psychiatry*, 55, S379-84.

Hariprasad, V. R., Koparde, V., Sivakumar, P. T., Varambally, S., Thirthalli, J., Varghese, M., Basavaraddi, I. V. & Gangadhar, B. N. (2013b). Randomized clinical trial of yoga-based intervention in residents from elderly homes: effects on cognitive function. *Indian J Psychiatry*, 55, S357-63.

Hariprasad, V. R., Varambally, S., Shivakumar, V., Kalmady, S. V., Venkatasubramanian, G. & Gangadhar, B. N. (2013c). Yoga increases the volume of the hippocampus in elderly subjects. *Indian J Psychiatry*, 55, S394-6.

Hassasiri, A., Dhammakhanto, K. & Wongpunya, S. (2002). Manual of meditation and imagery training for attention deficit children: age 5–11. *8th International Congress of Department of Mental Health*. Thailand.

Hegarty, J. D., Baldessarini, R. J., Tohen, M., Waternaux, C. & Oepen, G. (1994). One hundred years of schizophrenia: a meta-analysis of the outcome literature. *Am J Psychiatry*, 151, 1409–16.

Hofer, A., Benecke, C., Edlinger, M., Huber, R., Kemmler, G., Rettenbacher, M. A., Schleich, G. & Wolfgang Fleischhacker, W. (2009). Facial emotion recognition and its relationship to symptomatic, subjective, and functional outcomes in outpatients with chronic schizophrenia. *Eur Psychiatry*, 24, 27–32.

Iyengar, B. K. (1966). *Light on Yoga.*, New Delhi, Harper Collins India.

Janakiramaiah, N., Gangadhar, B. N., Naga venkatesha murthy, P. J., Harish, M. G., Subbakrishna, D. K. & Vedamurthachar, A. (2000). Antidepressant efficacy of Sudarshan Kriya Yoga (SKY) in melancholia: a randomized comparison with electroconvulsive therapy (ECT) and imipramine. *J Affect Disord*, 57, 255–9.

Jayaram, N., Varambally, S., Behere, R. V., Venkatasubramanian, G., Arasappa, R., Christopher, R. & Gangadhar, B. N. (2013). Effect of yoga therapy on plasma oxytocin and facial emotion recognition deficits in patients of schizophrenia. *Indian J Psychiatry*, 55, S409-13.

Jensen, P. S. & Kenny, D. T. (2004). The effects of yoga on the attention and behavior of boys with attention-deficit/ hyperactivity disorder (ADHD). *J Atten Disord*, 7, 205–16.

John, P. J., Sharma, N., Sharma, C. M. & Kankane, A. (2007) Effectiveness of yoga therapy in the treatment of migraine without aura: a randomized controlled trial. *Headache*, 47, 654–61.

Kabat-Zinn, J., Massion, A. O., Kristeller, J., Peterson, L. G., Fletcher, K. E., Pbert, L., Lenderking, W. R. & Santorelli, S. F. (1992). Effectiveness of a meditation-based stress reduction program in the treatment of anxiety disorders. *Am J Psychiatry*, 149, 936–43.

Kay, S., Fiszbein, A. & Opler, R. (1987). The positive and negative syndrome scale for schizophrenia (PANSS). *Schizophr Bull*, 261–76.

Kee, K. S., Green, M. F., Mintz, J. & Brekke, J. S. (2003). Is emotion processing a predictor of functional outcome in schizophrenia? *Schizophr Bull*, 29, 487–97.

Kessler, R. C., Soukup, J., Davis, R. B., Foster, D. F., Wilkey, S. A., Van Rompay, M. I. & Eisenberg, D. M. (2001). The use of complementary and alternative therapies to treat anxiety and depression in the United States. *Am J Psychiatry*, 158, 289–94.

Khalsa, S. B. (2004) Treatment of chronic insomnia with yoga: a preliminary study with sleep-wake diaries. *Appl Psychophysiol Biofeedback*, 29, 269–78.

Khalsa, S. B., Khalsa, G. S., Khalsa, H. K. & Khalsa, M. K. (2008). Evaluation of a residential Kundalini yoga lifestyle pilot program for addiction in India. *J Ethn Subst Abuse*, 7, 67–79.

Khanna, S. & Greeson, J. M. (2013). A narrative review of yoga and mindfulness as complementary therapies for addiction. *Complement Ther Med*, 21, 244–52.

Khumar, S. S., Kaur, P. & Kaur, S. (1993) Effectiveness of Shavasana on depression among university students. *Indian J Clin Psychol*, 20, 82–87.

Kirkwood, G., Rampes, H., Tuffrey, V., Richardson, J. & Pilkington, K. (2005). Yoga for anxiety: a systematic review of the research evidence. *Br J Sports Med*, 39, 884–91, discussion 891.

Kisan, R., Sujan, M., Adoor, M., Rao, R., Nalini, A., Kutty, B. M., Chindanda Murthy, B., Raju, T. & Sathyaprabha, T. (2014) Effect of Yoga on migraine: A comprehensive study using clinical profile and cardiac autonomic functions. *Int J Yoga*, 7, 126–32.

Kochupillai, V., Kumar, P., Singh, D., Aggarwal, D., Bhardwaj, N., Bhutani, M. & Das, S. N. (2005). Effect of rhythmic breathing (Sudarshan Kriya and Pranayam) on immune functions and tobacco addiction. *Ann N Y Acad Sci*, 1056, 242–52.

Kozasa, E. H., Santos, R. F., Rueda, A. D., Benedito-Silva, A. A., De Ornellas, F. L. & Leite, J. R. (2008). Evaluation of Siddha Samadhi Yoga for anxiety and depression symptoms: a preliminary study. *Psychol Rep*, 103, 271–4.

Krisanaprakornkit, T., Ngamjarus, C., Witoonchart, C. & Piyavhatkul, N. (2010). Meditation therapies for attention-deficit/hyperactivity disorder (ADHD). *Cochrane Database Syst Rev*, CD006507.

Krishnamurthy, M. N. & Telles, S. (2007). Assessing depression following two ancient Indian interventions: effects of yoga and ayurveda on older adults in a residential home. *J Gerontol Nurs*, 33, 17–23.

Langhorst, J., Klose, P., Dobos, G. J., Bernardy, K. & Hauser, W. (2013) Efficacy and safety of meditative movement therapies in fibromyalgia syndrome: a systematic review and meta-analysis of randomized controlled trials. *Rheumatol Int*, 33, 193–207.

Lazar, S. W., Kerr, C. E., Wasserman, R. H., Gray, J. R., Greve, D. N., Treadway, M. T., Mcgarvey, M., Quinn, B. T., Dusek, J. A., Benson, H., Rauch, S. L.,

Moore, C. I. & Fischl, B. (2005). Meditation experience is associated with increased cortical thickness. *Neuroreport*, 16, 1893–7.

Luders, E., Toga, A. W., Lepore, N. & Gaser, C. (2009). The underlying anatomical correlates of long-term meditation: larger hippocampal and frontal volumes of gray matter. *Neuroimage*, 45, 672–8.

Manjunath, R. B., Varambally, S., Thirthalli, J., Basavaraddi, I. V. & Gangadhar, B. N. (2013) Efficacy of yoga as an add-on treatment for in-patients with functional psychotic disorder. *Indian J Psychiatry*, 55, S374–8.

Mehta, S., Mehta, V., Shah, D., Motiwala, A., Vardhan, J., Mehta, N. & Mehta, D. (2011). Multimodal behavior program for ADHD incorporating yoga and implemented by high school volunteers: a pilot study. *ISRN Pediatr*, 2011, 780745.

Mehta, S., Shah, D., Shah, K., Mehta, N., Mehta, V., Motiwala, S. & Mehta, D. (2013). Peer-mediated multimodal intervention program for the treatment of children with ADHD in India: one-year followup. *ISRN Pediatr*, 2012, 419168.

Mist, S. D., Firestone, K. A. & Jones, K. D. (2013) Complementary and alternative exercise for fibromyalgia: a meta-analysis. *J Pain Res*, 6, 247–60.

Moretti-Altuna, G. E. (1987) *The effects of meditation versus medication in the treatment of attention deficit disorder with hyperactivity.* Department of Psychology New York, at St. John's University.

Murthy, P. J., Gangadhar, B. N., Janakiramaiah, N. & Subbakrishna, D. K. (1997). Normalization of P300 amplitude following treatment in dysthymia. *Biol Psychiatry*, 42, 740–3.

Mustian, K. M., Sprod, L. K., Janelsins, M., Peppone, L. J., Palesh, O. G., Chandwani, K., Reddy, P. S., Melnik, M. K., Heckler, C. & Morrow, G. R. (2013) Multicenter, randomized controlled trial of yoga for sleep quality among cancer survivors. *J Clin Oncol*, 31, 3233–41.

Nagendra, H. R., Telles, S., Naveen, K V. (2000). An integrated approach of Yoga therapy for the management of schizophrenia. Final Report submitted to Dept. of ISM & H, Ministry of Health and Family Welfare, Government of India, New Delhi

Naveen, G. H., Rao, M. G., Vishal, V., Thirthalli, J., Varambally, S. & Gangadhar, B. N. (2013a). Development and feasibility of yoga therapy module for out-patients with depression in India. *Indian J Psychiatry*, 55, S350-6.

Naveen, G. H., Thirthalli, J., Rao, M. G., Varambally, S., Christopher, R. & Gangadhar, B. N. (2013b). Positive therapeutic and neurotropic effects of yoga in depression: a comparative study. *Indian J Psychiatry*, 55, S400-4.

Norton, G. R. & Johnson, W. E. (1983). A comparison of two relaxation procedures for reducing cognitive and somatic anxiety. *J Behav Ther Exp Psychiatry*, 14, 209–14.

Ong, J. C., Shapiro, S. L. & Manber, R. (2008) Combining mindfulness meditation with cognitive-behavior therapy for insomnia: a treatment-development study. *Behav Ther*, 39, 171–82.

Patra, S. & Telles, S. (2009) Positive impact of cyclic meditation on subsequent sleep. *Med Sci Monit*, 15, CR375–81.

Pilkington, K., Kirkwood, G., Rampes, H. & Richardson, J. (2005). Yoga for depression: the research evidence. *J Affect Disord*, 89, 13–24.

Rani, K., Tiwari, S. C., Singh, U., Agrawal, G. G. & Srivastava, N. (2011) Six-month trial of Yoga Nidra in menstrual disorder patients: Effects on somatoform symptoms. *Ind Psychiatry J*, 20, 97–102.

Ravindran, A. V. & Da Silva, T. L. (2013). Complementary and alternative therapies as add-on to pharmacotherapy for mood and anxiety disorders: a systematic review. *J Affect Disord*, 150, 707–19.

Ravindran, A. V., Lam, R. W., Filteau, M. J., Lesperance, F., Kennedy, S. H., Parikh, S. V. & Patten, S. B. (2009). Canadian Network for Mood and Anxiety Treatments (CANMAT) Clinical guidelines for the management of major depressive disorder in adults. V. Complementary and alternative medicine treatments. *J Affect Disord*, 117 (Suppl 1), S54–64.

Saraswat, N., Rao, K., Subbakrishna, D. K. & Gangadhar, B. N. (2006). The Social Occupational Functioning Scale (SOFS): a brief measure of functional status in persons with schizophrenia. *Schizophr Res*, 81, 301–9.

Selye, H. (1956). Stress and psychiatry. *Am J Psychiatry*, 113, 423–27.

Shaffer, H. J., Lasalvia, T. A. & Stein, J. P. (1997). Comparing Hatha yoga with dynamic group psychotherapy for enhancing methadone maintenance treatment: a randomized clinical trial. *Altern Ther Health Med*, 3, 57–66.

Shannahoff-Khalsa, D. S. & Beckett, L. R. (1996). Clinical case report: efficacy of yogic techniques in the treatment of obsessive compulsive disorders. *Int J Neurosci*, 85, 1–17.

Shannahoff-Khalsa, D. S., Ray, L. E., Levine, S., Gallen, C. C., Schwartz, B. J. & Sidorowich, J. J. (1999). Randomized controlled trial of yogic meditation techniques for patients with obsessive-compulsive disorder. *CNS Spectr*, 4, 34–47.

Shapiro, D., Cook, I. A., Davydov, D. M., Ottaviani, C., Leuchter, A. F. & Abrams, M. (2007). Yoga as a complementary treatment of depression: effects of traits and moods on treatment outcome. *Evid Based Complement Alternat Med*, 4, 493–502.

Sharma, I., Azmi, S. A. & Settiwar, R. M. (1991). Evaluation of the effect of pranayama in anxiety state. *Altern. Med.*, 3 (4), 227–35

Sharma, V. K., Das, S., Mondal, S., Goswampi, U. & Gandhi, A. (2005). Effect of sahaj yoga on depressive disorders. *Indian J Physiol Pharmacol*, 49, 462–8.

Sharma, V. K., Das, S., Mondal, S., Goswami, U. & Gandhi, A. (2006). Effect of sahaj yoga on neuro-cognitive functions in patients suffering from major depression. *Indian J Physiol Pharmacol*, 50, 375–83.

Sherman, T., Mueser, K. T., Osborne, D. D., Currier, M. & Wolfe, R. (2005). The effects of yoga on mood in psychiatric inpatients. *Psychiatr Rehabil J*, 28, 399–402.

Streeter, C. C., Jensen, J. E., Perlmutter, R. M., Cabral, H. J., Tian, H., Terhune, D. B., Ciraulo, D. A. & Renshaw, P. F. (2007). Yoga Asana sessions increase brain GABA levels: a pilot study. *J Altern Complement Med*, 13, 419–26.

Streeter, C. C., Whitfield, T. H., Owen, L., Rein, T., Karri, S. K., Yakhkind, A., Perlmutter, R., Prescot, A., Renshaw, P. F., Ciraulo, D. A. & Jensen, J. E. (2010). Effects of yoga versus walking on mood, anxiety, and brain GABA levels: a randomized controlled MRS study. *J Altern Complement Med*, 16, 1145–52.

Sutar, R. (2014) Effect of yoga intervention in patients with somatoform disorders: A pilot study. *Psychiatry*. Bangalore, National Institute of Mental Health and Neurosciences.

Tyagi, A. & Cohen, M. (2014). Yoga and hypertension: a systematic review. *Altern Ther Health Med*, 20, 32–59.

Uebelacker, L. A., Epstein-Lubow, G., Gaudiano, B. A., Tremont, G., Battle, C. L. & Miller, I. W. (2010). Hatha yoga for depression: critical review of the evidence for efficacy, plausible mechanisms of action, and directions for future research. *J Psychiatr Pract*, 16, 22–33.

Varambally, S., Behere, R., Thirthalli, J., Duraiswamy, G., Arasappa, R., Venkatasubramanian, G. & Gangadhar, B. N. (2010). Yoga for the negative symptoms of schizophrenia: new promise from an ancient science. *Australian and New Zealand Journal of psychiatry*, 44, A36.

Varambally, S. & Gangadhar, B. N. (2012). Yoga: a spiritual practice with therapeutic value in psychiatry. *Asian J Psychiatr*, 5, 186–9.

Varambally, S., Gangadhar, B. N., Thirthalli, J., Jagannathan, A., Kumar, S., Venkatasubramanian, G., Muralidhar, D., Subbakrishna, D. K. & Nagendra, H. R. (2012). Therapeutic efficacy of add-on yogasana intervention in stabilized outpatient schizophrenia: randomized controlled comparison with exercise and wait-list. *Indian J Psychiatry*, 54, 227–32.

Vedamurthachar, A., Janakiramaiah, N., Hegde, J. M., Shetty, T. K., Subbakrishna, D. K., Sureshbabu, S. V. & Gangadhar, B. N. (2006). Antidepressant efficacy and hormonal effects of Sudarshana Kriya Yoga (SKY) in alcohol dependent individuals. *J Affect Disord*, 94, 249–53.

Visceglia, E. & Lewis, S. (2011). Yoga therapy as an adjunctive treatment for schizophrenia: a randomized, controlled pilot study. *J Altern Complement Med*, 17, 601–7.

Voineskos, D., Rogasch, N. C., Rajji, T. K., Fitzgerald, P. B. & Daskalakis, Z. J. (2013). A review of evidence linking disrupted neural plasticity to schizophrenia. *Can J Psychiatry*, 58, 86–92.

Vollestad, J., Nielsen, M. B. & Nielsen, G. H. (2012). Mindfulness- and acceptance-based interventions for anxiety disorders: a systematic review and meta-analysis. *Br J Clin Psychol*, 51, 239–60.

Vollestad, J., Sivertsen, B. & Nielsen, G. H. (2011). Mindfulness-based stress reduction for patients with anxiety disorders: evaluation in a randomized controlled trial. *Behav Res Ther*, 49, 281–8.

Walsh, R. & Roche, L. (1979). Precipitation of acute psychotic episodes by intensive meditation in individuals with a history of schizophrenia. *Am J Psychiatry*, 136, 1085–6.

Woolery, A., Myers, H., Sternlieb, B. & Zeltzer, L. (2004). A yoga intervention for young adults with elevated symptoms of depression. *Altern Ther Health Med*, 10, 60–3.

10

Physical exercise for brain health in later life: how does it work?

Amit Lampit, Shantel L. Duffy and Michael Valenzuela

Physical inactivity is the most prevalent dementia risk factor in developed countries, associated with an 86% increased risk of Alzheimer's disease (AD) as well as other chronic conditions such as cardiovascular disease, obesity and diabetes (Norton et al., 2014). Human studies indicate that increased physical activity and exercise are effective at improving cognitive function in older adults, but the mechanisms underlying these effects are just beginning to be understood. Promotion of physical exercise therefore has great potential as a risk reduction strategy, and a better biological understanding of its therapeutic basis could aid development of even more effective interventions and inform practice, as well as improve our understanding of the brain's plastic potential and limits. That said, to date there has been insufficient recognition of the fundamental differences in research outcomes in animals and humans, simplistic extrapolations from one to the other and gaps in our knowledge. In this chapter, we briefly review these issues and ask whether this disconnect could be hampering successful backwards and forwards translation in this area.

Physical exercise, cognition and dementia in late life: what do clinical studies tell us about possible mechanisms?

A valuable distinction in the human clinical literature is whether the object of investigation is incremental change on one or more cognitive outcomes (i.e., continuous variables) or categorical health-related outcomes such as dementia prevalence or incidence (binary variables) or daily function (ordinal variable). This has large implications on the design of studies and their end significance. Sensitive measures of cognition can readily detect change over a relatively short period of time but have limited relevance to real-life outcomes (Salthouse, 2012)

Physical Exercise Interventions for Mental Health, ed. Linda C. W. Lam and Michelle Riba. Published by Cambridge University Press. © Cambridge University Press 2016.

or to socioeconomic models of disease burden. On the other hand, categorical health-related measures are of obvious personal and social significance, but these measures have low fidelity and are relatively insensitive to change, making their use in clinical research onerous in time and resources.

Epidemiological studies provide extensive evidence for a link between long-term patterns of physical activity and domains of cognition known to be susceptible to age-related decline. This includes associations between greater physical activity and lower rates of longitudinal decline on measures of global cognition (Yaffe et al., 2009) as well as specific cognitive domains. A recent meta-analysis of 15 longitudinal studies found decreased risk of cognitive decline (measured by an array of neuropsychological tests) of 38% and 35% in older people with high and moderate physical activity levels respectively, compared to those with low activity levels (Sofi et al., 2011). Whilst studies in this meta-analysis varied substantially methodologically, results were relatively homogenous, and these differences did not determine outcomes. Yet despite the number of studies, we still do not have good epidemiological evidence about which cognitive domains may be specifically protected by physical activity or are at-risk through inactivity. To the best of our knowledge, there is no meta-analysis of cohort studies of physical exercise and cognitive change that has specifically compared outcomes between cognitive domains in older adults, an important knowledge gap in the field.

Epidemiological studies also associate long-term patterns of physical activity with reduced risk of dementia. Barnes and Yaffe (2011) reviewed 16 cohort studies and found a 28% decreased risk for all-cause dementia and 45% reduction in AD dementia in those with higher activity levels compared to low. In addition, some individual studies indicate dose-dependency between levels of physical activity and relative risk reduction (Podewils et al., 2005; Scarmeas et al., 2009), suggesting that even small gains in activity may benefit older adults, irrespective of whether individuals reach official exercise recommendations (Sparling et al., 2015).

There is therefore a case that exercise may be useful as a means to better preserve cognition and prevent or delay dementia, at least at the population level, but several caveats need to be considered. Firstly, these studies rely on self-report of current or mid-life physical activity patterns, data that are prone to various forms of bias. Physical inactivity is also a risk factor for many other conditions that may affect cognition and elevate AD risk, and so the unique variance attributable to activity is challenging to precisely estimate (Norton et al., 2014). Moreover, it is in principle impossible to control for the full suite of relevant variables that covary with physical activity because of factors that we do not know about, and the possibility of reverse causality is difficult to exclude. For example, individuals with premorbid and undetected dementia may drop-off physical activity or selectively recall their past experiences in the lead-up to diagnosis, artificially producing an association at follow-up. Finally, a meta-regression analysis found no relationship between physical fitness and cognitive performance in cross-sectional studies, suggesting that the mechanism by which activity influences cognition may be independent of aerobic capacity *per se* (Etnier et al., 2006).

Randomised controlled trials (RCTs) of exercise interventions address many of the temporal primacy problems left hanging in epidemiological studies. Colcombe and Kramer (2003) identified 18 RCTs of exercise in older adults, and found a large effect size on executive processes ($g = 0.68$), as well as small effect sizes on controlled ($g = 0.17$) and speed ($g = 0.27$) tasks, but no effect on memory. Importantly, cognitive effects were greater in studies that combined strength and aerobic exercise, and were substantially smaller when sessions were shorter than 30 minutes. More recently, Smith and colleagues (2010) reviewed 29 RCTs of aerobic or combined exercise, 22 in older adults. Once again, significant effects were noted for executive function, attention and processing speed, but effect sizes were small ($g < 0.2$). A small effect size was also found for memory but not on working memory, although combined interventions did seem to be efficacious on this domain. Finally, a meta-analysis designed specifically to examine exercise and memory (Roig et al., 2013) found that only *acute* exercise (i.e., a total dose ranging from 30 seconds to 65 minutes) improved performance on short- and long-term memory tasks, whereas *long-term* exercise (i.e., the subject of RCTs) produced a substantially smaller effect size on short-term memory ($g = 0.15$) and no effect on long-term memory.

In summary, physical activity and long-term exercise interventions could be beneficial for maintaining cognition and preventing or delaying dementia onset in the community. However, the biological mechanisms may be at least partly independent of aerobic fitness, and indirect pathways via attenuation of co-morbid systemic diseases also known to affect cognition cannot be ruled out. The RCT literature in older adults demonstrates that long-term exercise interventions produce modest effect sizes on cognition, with more consistent evidence for efficacy on frontal-executive function and limited evidence for efficacy on memory.

Animal models of exercise: what is and is not relevant to humans?

Several comprehensive reviews of the effects of exercise on the rodent brain are available elsewhere (e.g., Prakash et al., 2015; Voss et al., 2013a) and not replicated here. These reviews are hippocentric – focusing extensively on evidence for molecular, trophic and cellular plasticity in the hippocampus. Rather, in this section we focus on animal evidence for exercise-dependent frontal-executive plasticity, the result with most convincing human clinical data. However, prior to this it is instructive to highlight some issues that complicate direct and simplistic extrapolation of animal exercise research into insights about human biology.

Enrichment versus exercise

Many animal studies of physical exercise are in fact environmental enrichment studies, where the animal is exposed to a multifactorial change in living conditions with not only additional opportunities for physical exercise (typically by introducing a running wheel), but also for social interaction (via bigger cages and new littermates) and cognitive stimulation (via exploration of new objects including the running wheel itself) (Nithianantharajah and Hannan, 2006).

At this time, it is not clear which cluster of neurobiological mechanisms triggered by voluntary running is unique and distinct to those triggered by environmental enrichment, with some interesting recent studies attempting to dissociate these factors (Cracchiolo et al., 2007; Smith et al., 2013) The implication of this is that many of the mechanisms suggested to be dependent on physical exercise are, in fact, dependent on a multimodal intervention that often includes social and cognitive stimulation. From a translation point of view, this is not a major problem because even the most rigorous physical exercise RCT in humans will require additional social and cognitive stimulation because of the nature of trial participation. Nevertheless, it is worthwhile to consider the degree of modality specificity when evaluating animal studies of exercise.

Control housing as solitary confinement

Control housing in rodent studies of exercise comprises either individual housing or small group housing (1–2 other animals) in a static unchanging world. Bedding (e.g., shredded newspaper) and feed do not change, and the only likely break from this monotony is an occasional check by the animal assistant (which animals tend to anticipate and react inquisitively to over time). By comparison, the natural environment of a rodent is complex, social, changing and considerably more challenging to live and survive in.

An often-neglected translational issue is therefore that control housing in animal exercise experiments is more akin to a human gaol – and in the case of single-housing more like solitary confinement. Indeed, most gaols in developed countries allow their inmates some degree of physical exercise *ad libitum*. The impact of the introduction of running wheels into an experimental rodent's physical world cannot therefore be underestimated. The degree of behavioural change is drastic – in our study of aged rats, voluntary movement increased from a matter of centimeters per day (in fact per night) to about 200m per night (Siette et al., 2013). It is then perhaps not surprising that such a broad range of metabolic, trophic, transcriptional, cellular, network changes are found in these animals. The correct analogy is perhaps inmates in solitary confinement for most of their life suddenly being allowed to exercise freely at a gym. Clearly, no human trial has that kind of dynamic range, and so the mechanisms observed in animal studies must be thought of as potential maxima rather than likely in humans. This is perhaps just one reason why the startling finding that voluntary running is capable of substantially decreasing Alzheimer's disease plaques in (some strains of) transgenic mice (Lazarov et al., 2005) has yet to be replicated in humans (Bennett et al., 2014).

Dosage and lifespan exposures

The great majority of animal studies of exercise commence the intervention post weaning (>3 months age), intervene for a matter of weeks or months and then sacrifice the animal. These are therefore studies of the effect of exercise during a large part of the adult animal's life. By contrast, studies where exercise commences in aged animals are uncommon (Siette et al., 2013; van Praag et al., 2005) but much more relevant to human health since this is the general target of 'early intervention trials'. We therefore know much less about the neurobiological effects of voluntary running in the aged rodent brain than in the adult rodent brain.

Wheel running versus lifting weights

Animal models of physical exercise are almost exclusively models of aerobic exercise and, more specifically, voluntary running. Rodents naturally run from a to b, so immediately there is a translational challenge when attempting to equate voluntary running in mice and men (and women). Most RCTs in the elderly are also based on mild-to-moderate increases in exercise such as increased walking; to take one successful example, Lautenschlager et al. (2008) found a small positive effect on global cognition (approximately 1 ADAS-COG point change difference) in their exercise group, attributed to a behavioural change in participants of approximately 9000 steps per week, a 16% increase in the number of walked steps. We are not aware of any animal study that has modelled the neurobiological impact of a 10–20% increase in baseline voluntary running, movement or behaviour.

More and more human studies suggest that resistance exercise may produce unique modulatory effects on inflammatory cascades that are directly relevant to brain biology (Strasser and Pesta, 2013), as well as protecting cognitive (Fiatarone Singh et al., 2014) and brain (Liu-Ambrose et al., 2012) function. To date, there is a dearth of animal models of resistance exercise and very few that have linked neurobiological and cognitive changes to resistance exercise in rodents (Cassilhas et al., 2012).

Comorbid disease outcomes

Epidemiological studies indicate that at least some of the links between physical activity and cognitive health may be attributable to reduced risk for metabolic (diabetes, obesity, hyperlidemia) and vascular disease (hypertension, coronary artery disease and cerebrovascular disease). Indeed, there is a growing awareness of the contribution of these chronic disorders, particularly hypertension and cerebrovascular disease, to cognition and dementia risk in late life (Valenzuela et al., 2012).

Animal models of the neurobiological effects of exercise have essentially ignored this issue, with one notable exception. Several studies have shown that voluntary running induces angiogenesis (Bloor, 2005; van Praag et al., 2005) and vascular remodelling in the brain (Lopez-Lopez et al., 2004), with IGF-1 and VEGF likely to play roles in this process (Fabel et al., 2003). These mechanisms are certainly relevant to humans, to some extent verified in human studies using MR techniques to probe cerebral blood flow (Burdette et al., 2010), cerebral blood volume (Pereira et al., 2007) and vessel architecture (Bullitt et al., 2009). However, aged rodents do not naturally develop white matter ischemia and leukoaraiosis – markers of small vessel disease that contributes to fronto-executive dysfunction in human ageing and cognitive impairment (Debette and Markus, 2010; Pantoni, 2010) and, moreover, are likely to be responsive to physical exercise (Richard et al., 2010). A lack of understanding of the basic biological processes that may mediate these outcomes is therefore a major omission, a missing link with direct real-world relevance to human therapeutic efficacy.

Animal research standards

A "metachallenge" for animal bioscience is that the same standards for reporting RCTs in humans do not apply (see Special series in Nature, 2014). Hence, investigators do not need to stipulate primary or secondary outcomes in advance, register an experimental design or even account for the animals at the beginning, middle and end of the experiment. The problem of "the missing animals" is only beginning to be highlighted (see Begley, 2013) – it is common practice for one or more animals to be excluded from an analysis because 'it did not behave properly', a kind of adherence problem where the solution is simple: pretend it did not exist. In RCTs, intention-to-treat analyses are the gold standard, and it is well known that analysis of 'completers' can severely distort outcomes in favour of the investigators (Molnar et al., 2008). Why the same should not apply to experimental medicine has no defence (Landis et al., 2012). Lack of rigorous governance and reporting standard in the animal biosciences therefore calls into question many findings – systematic attempts to replicate high-profile animal studies have reported a > 70% failure rate (Prinz et al., 2011). Standards in the animal exercise literature is of course no exception; however, it should be emphasized that many of the high-profile hippocampal plasticity findings are robust and have been replicated in many labs around the world.

Exercise-dependent fronto-executive plasticity in rodents

With the caveats above in mind, we now turn to studies that have explored fronto-executive function in rodents in response to exercise. In rodents, this translates to studies of response speed, complex motor function, attention and problem solving. There are, in fact, very few studies. Early work showed that both short-term exercise (Meeusen et al., 1997) and long-term exercise (MacRae et al., 1987) increase monoamines in the striatum, a hypothetical basis for improved motor speed and co-ordination and, more speculatively, for cognitive speed. The importance of these neurotransmitters in potentially mediating exercise effects on frontal lobe function is further supported by two complementary studies. On the one hand, rodent models of ADHD have found that physical exercise can be as effective as drug treatment for the normalisation of orientating behaviour and social interaction (Robinson et al., 2012). On the other hand, selective breeding of mice that strongly exhibit running behaviour produces a pedigree of avid runners who are generally more active, spend less time inactive or grooming or sleeping, and have lower concentrations of key monoamines, such as dopamine and serotonin in the substantia nigra and dorsolateral putamen – evidence of a hypoactive nigro-striatal system that resembles human ADHD (Waters et al., 2013). Another potential biological mechanism for improved motor and cognitive speed after chronic exercise is a significant increase in mitochondrial biogenesis in the brain (Steiner et al., 2011); however, behavioural-pathological correlation studies have yet to establish a link. Altogether, there is a suggestion that monoaminergic adaptation of the nigro-striatal system may be implicated in exercise-induced improvements in frontal-executive function, but to date there has been insufficient animal research in this area.

Human studies of exercise-dependent frontal executive plasticity

There is extensive human evidence from neuroimaging studies that physical activity and exercise is linked to adaptation of brain structure and function. In general, the strongest effects are seen in those areas most likely to atrophy with age, including the frontal, temporal and parietal regions (Kirk-Sanchez and McGough, 2014; Prakash et al., 2015). These studies give important insights into the nature and limits of the human brain's plasticity in response to physical exercise, but because the spatial resolution of modern brain imaging techniques are in the mm range, the precise biological mechanisms cannot be defined.

Several neuroimaging studies demonstrate a longitudinal relationship between physical activity levels and brain atrophy in older adults. In a study conducted by Bugg and Head (2011), higher estimates of exercise engagement over the previous 10-year period moderated age-related medial temporal lobe atrophy and were correlated to greater frontal lobe volume. A subgroup analysis (n = 75) of a large population-based longitudinal study also found that individuals who engage in more physical activity in mid-life had larger frontal lobe volumes in later life compared with their more sedentary counterparts (Rovio et al., 2010). Similar results were also reported in the Cardiovascular Health Study (Erickson et al., 2010), which examined the association between grey matter volume, physical activity and cognition in 299 older adults over 9 years. Overall, higher levels of physical activity at baseline predicted larger frontal, occipital and medial temporal lobe volumes at follow up. Furthermore, greater grey matter volume was associated with a twofold reduction in risk for cognitive impairment at 13-years post baseline assessment.

These studies suggest that individual differences in long-term patterns of physical activity may have significant implications for regional brain volume and atrophy in later life. However, the same limitations apply as for epidemiological studies of exercise and cognitive risk. Specifically, these studies rely on self-reported physical activity rather than objective measures, severely limiting the ability to assess dose-response relationships (Erickson et al., 2012a). On the other hand, cross-sectional studies examining the relationship between objective measures of current cardiorespiratory fitness and brain volume point to similar results. A study examining 165 older adults showed that higher aerobic fitness is associated with greater hippocampal volume and, further, demonstrated that hippocampal volume mediates the relationship between aerobic fitness and memory function in older adults (Erickson et al., 2009). Of particular significance, aerobic capacity is also related to brain volume in patients with cognitive impairment. For example, larger total grey matter volume and medial temporal lobe volume have been demonstrated in AD patients with higher levels of aerobic fitness (Honea et al., 2009). But regional brain changes linked with physical activity are not only restricted to the medial temporal lobe, with cross-sectional research also connecting physical activity with prefrontal cortex volume and executive function (Erickson et al., 2012a; Kirk-Sanchez and McGough, 2014; Prakash et al., 2015). For example, a study conducted by Colcombe and colleagues (2003) demonstrated that greater cardiorespiratory fitness is associated with greater prefrontal cortex volume in community-dwelling older adults. Weinstein and colleagues (2012) further showed that prefrontal cortex volume mediates the relationship between executive function and cardiorespiratory fitness in older adults. Yet, as reviewed above, a large meta-regression has failed to establish a link between individual differences in cardiac fitness and cognitive function in older adults (Etnier et al., 2006), suggesting that whilst aerobic fitness may be an important correlate of prefrontal volume it is not necessarily relevant to cognition in general.

Once again, RCT designs are particularly valuable at decomposing long-term brain-behaviour dependencies seen in observational studies into cause-and-effect. An RCT by Colcombe and colleagues (2006) using voxel-based morphometry found attenuation of atrophy and even trophic gains in regional brain volumes in a group of sedentary older adults randomised to a six-month walking intervention compared to a stretching control group. Specific increases were found in the anterior cingulate cortex, dorsolateral prefrontal cortex and temporal lobe, as well as increased volume of the anterior white matter tracts. However, not all studies have replicated these findings. Ruscheweyh and colleagues (2011) examined the effect of a moderate-intensity walking intervention, a low-intensity stretching intervention and a control intervention in inactive older adults and found no difference in brain structure between groups. Similarly, Voss and colleagues (2013a) demonstrated no between-group changes in white matter integrity following a 12-months moderate-intensity walking intervention. On the other hand, both studies demonstrated that changes in grey and white matter correlated with improved cardiorespiratory fitness in the aerobic exercise groups. Accordingly, these findings suggest that improvement in fitness levels rather than simple participation in physical activity interventions may be required to elicit changes in brain structure and, furthermore, that the extent of fitness gains in these RCTs may have been insufficient to produce detectable changes in brain volume.

Dynamical changes in brain function linked to exercise have also been investigated using functional Magnetic Resonance Imaging (fMRI; Prakash et al., 2015). In two cross-sectional studies conducted by Colcombe and colleagues (2004), highly fit or aerobically trained individuals exhibited greater activity in parietal and prefrontal regions in response to executive function tasks when compared to individuals with low levels of fitness or those in a control condition. Similarly, Prakash and colleagues (2011) found increased prefrontal cortical recruitment during a complex response inhibition task in older adults with greater cardiorespiratory fitness. Using an RCT design, Colcombe and colleagues (2004) documented increased frontal and parietal activation and reduced anterior cingulate cortex recruitment during the performance of a different response inhibition task following a six-month aerobic exercise intervention. Physical activity has also been shown to improve spontaneous or resting-state network synchrony in aged individuals. Whilst the default mode network and the frontal-executive networks typically demonstrate age-related desynchronisation, a 12-month walking intervention resulted in increased functional connectivity in both these networks, also associated with improved executive functioning (Voss et al., 2010). All these findings therefore converge on the notion that moderate-intensity aerobic exercise can trigger positive adaptation of task-based and resting-state prefrontal cortical networks in older adults. Importantly, this conclusion is supported by evidence from another imaging modality, magnetic resonance spectroscopy. Erickson and colleagues (2012b) showed in a cross-sectional study that higher levels of aerobic fitness attenuated age-related decline in a key neuronal-specific metabolite, N-acetyl aspartate, specifically in the frontal lobe.

In summary, long-term patterns of physical activity are related to a broad range of structural brain difference in late life, especially in the frontal cortex and medial temporal lobe. Cardiorespiratory fitness may mediate these linkages; however, this does not necessary help explain variability in late-life cognitive function. Structural findings from RCT-based imaging studies have not been well replicated; however, fMRI studies clearly identify prefrontal cortex as a focus of aerobic exercise-induced plasticity with relevance to executive function.

A critical examination of medial temporal lobe plasticity in older humans

Given the mass of animal literature supporting multifactorial exercise-induced plastic mechanisms in the hippocampus relevant to performance on memory, learning and spatial navigation tasks, it is worthwhile to critically examine whether similar processes are relevant in humans, particularly older humans.

As reviewed above, there is only weak evidence that commencing an aerobic physical exercise program in late life is effective at protecting or improving memory. At best, the effect size is so small as to be clinically uninteresting. One caveat here is the possibility that the most sensitive memory tests have not been applied. Animal exercise studies indicate that adult hippocampal neurogenesis is reliably and robustly stimulated (Voss et al., 2013a), and it is claimed that spatial pattern separation is the most faithful behavioural correlate of this process in rodents (Clelland et al., 2009; Sahay et al., 2011), despite some controversy (Groves et al., 2013). Human neuropsychological versions of pattern separation are now available (Stark et al., 2010) and are sensitive to age-related decline (Holden et al., 2012), and so whether these cognitive tests would be more sensitive to physical exercise than traditional memory tests is an interesting question.

Rather, as reviewed above, the most consistent links between physical exercise, cardiovascular fitness and the medial temporal lobe have come from observational studies employing structural MRI. A number of studies have reported a protective link (Bugg and Head, 2011; Erickson et al., 2009; Erickson et al., 2010; Honea et al., 2009). What then is the functional relevance of this observation, if any? Clearly, the most accurate insight must come from studies employing an RCT-type design. Four such studies have now investigated the impact of aerobic exercise. Two have failed to report structural hippocampal plasticity (Ruscheweyh et al., 2011; Voss et al., 2013a), and two from the same group have reported positive outcomes (Colcombe et al., 2006; Erickson et al., 2011). The most recent and high-profile study (Erickson et al., 2011) reported a 2% increase in hippocampal volume in those who underwent a 12-month aerobic exercise intervention, compared to a 1.5% decline in volume in the control group (a net effect size of $d = 0.21$). Critically, this study employed a surface-based approach to model hippocampal shape and volume (the FSL FIRST procedure) and did not employ gold-standard expert tracing of the hippocampus. It is well known that findings of structural plasticity in the brain can be highly pipeline-dependent (Valenzuela et al., 2011), and so without corroboration by an independent analytical method it is hard to evaluate their biological significance. Beyond the small and unreplicated structural effects in the hippocampus, this same study did not find a significant improvement in memory. As publicly criticised (Coen et al., 2011), the title of the paper declared a positive effect on memory, but there was, in fact, no significant difference in spatial memory performance in those who undertook the aerobic intervention (2.3% accuracy improvement) compared to the stretching control (3.5% improvement), despite a net gain in cardiac fitness of 6.7%. Hence, even if one were to take the structural hippocampal findings at face value, these did not predict or explain any meaningful change in memory performance. It is also interesting to note that of all the fMRI studies to examine aerobic exercise (reviewed above), none have reported plasticity of hippocampal networks, a change likely to be necessary for therapeutic mnemonic outcomes.

The current state of the literature is therefore that unlike rodents, aerobic physical intervention does not produce consistent therapeutic benefits to memory, but like rodents, positive long-term physical activity patterns are linked to detectable difference in hippocampal volume that are in the opposite direction to ageing and early AD. Accordingly, in RCTs either the biological effects in the hippocampus are so weak as to be functionally irrelevant, or the functional biology of memory in humans does not map well onto rodent neuroscience. In either case, there is a translational gap.

Conclusions

Our understanding of the mechanisms by which physical exercise promotes and protects human cognitive function is rudimentary. The bulk of this knowledge comes from animal studies that are highly focused on hippocampal biology. These suggest that even a short period of voluntary wheel running can trigger a cascade of neurobiological effects at different spatial and temporal scales, but the relevance of this knowledge to humans is unclear. Firstly, several fundamental issues limit direct translation of animal research of aerobic exercise to humans. Not least is the basic issue that human RCTs typically involve incremental increases in natural physical activity (e.g., a little extra walking each day) compared to the quantum shift in exercise patterns typically modelled in rodents. Secondly, in humans the most consistent therapeutic benefits for exercise is in the domain of fronto-executive function, supported by evidence of adaptation of frontal lobe cortical networks, but the rodent literature has largely ignored this in favour of investigation of medial temporal lobe changes and memory. By contrast, human memory performance is only marginally affected by physical exercise interventions, and direct evidence for hippocampal structural plasticity remains unreplicated. A small number of animal studies suggest that exercise may trigger adaptation of nigrostriatal monoamine neurotransmitter systems, a finding with arguably more relevance to human cognitive health and one that merits more intensive research. Thirdly, human cognition in late life is affected by several co-morbid factors, not least cerebrovascular disease, known to directly impact fronto-executive function and to be sensitive to physical exercise patterns. The lack of rodent exercise research connecting chronic cerebrovascular disease with executive function is therefore yet another major gap in our understanding. All told, an unsatisfactory disconnect has emerged between clinical and epidemiological research on the one end and animal behavioural neuroscience on the other. For truly insightful advances in our understanding of how exercise benefits the human brain and cognitive health, better questions need to be traded backwards and forwards between researchers.

References

Barnes, D. E. & Yaffe, K. 2011. The projected effect of risk factor reduction on Alzheimer's disease prevalence. *Lancet Neurology*, 10, 819–28.

Begley, C. G. 2013. Six red flags for suspect work. *Nature*, 497, 433–4.

Bennett, D. A., Arnold, S. E., Valenzuela, M. J., Brayne, C. & Schneider, J. A. 2014. Cognitive and social lifestyle: links with neuropathology and cognition in late life. *Acta Neuropathologica*, 127, 137–50.

Bloor, C. M. 2005. Angiogenesis during exercise and training. *Angiogenesis*, 8, 263–71.

Bugg, J. M. & Head, D. 2011. Exercise moderates age-related atrophy of the medial temporal lobe. *Neurobiology of Aging*, 32, 506–14.

Bullitt, E., Ewend, M., Vredenburgh, J., Friedman, A., Lin, W., Wilber, K., Zeng, D., Aylward, S. R. & Reardon, D. 2009. Computerized assessment of vessel morphological changes during treatment of glioblastoma multiforme: report of a case imaged serially by MRA over four years. *Neuroimage*, 47 Suppl 2, T143–51.

Burdette, J. H., Laurienti, P. J., Espeland, M. A., Morgan, A., Telesford, Q., Vechlekar, C. D., Hayasaka, S., Jennings, J. M., Katula, J. A., Kraft, R. A. & Rejeski, W. J. 2010. Using network science to evaluate exercise-associated brain changes in older adults. *Frontiers in Aging Neuroscience*, 2, 23.

Cassilhas, R. C., Lee, K. S., Fernandes, J., Oliveira, M. G., Tufik, S., Meeusen, R. & De Mello, M. T. 2012. Spatial memory is improved by aerobic and resistance exercise through divergent molecular mechanisms. *Neuroscience*, 202, 309–17.

Clelland, C. D., Choi, M., Romberg, C., Clemenson, G. D., Jr., Fragniere, A., Tyers, P., Jessberger, S., Saksida, L. M., Barker, R. A., Gage, F. H. & Bussey, T. J. 2009. A functional role for adult hippocampal neurogenesis in spatial pattern separation. *Science*, 325, 210–3.

Coen, R. F., Lawlor, B. A. & Kenny, R. 2011. Failure to demonstrate that memory improvement is due either to aerobic exercise or increased hippocampal volume. *Proceedings of the National Academy of Sciences of the United States of America*, 108, E89; author reply E90.

Colcombe, S. J., Erickson, K. I., Raz, N., Webb, A. G., Cohen, N. J., McAuley, E. & Kramer, A. F. 2003. Aerobic fitness reduces brain tissue loss in aging humans. *Journals of Gerontology Series a: Biological Sciences and Medical Sciences*, 58, 176–80.

Colcombe, S. J., Erickson, K. I., Scalf, P. E., Kim, J. S., Prakash, R., McAuley, E., Elavsky, S., Marquez, D. X., Hu, L. & Kramer, A. F. 2006. Aerobic exercise training increases brain volume in aging humans. *Journals of Gerontology Series a: Biological Sciences and Medical Sciences*, 61, 1166–70.

Colcombe, S. & Kramer, A. F. 2003. Fitness effects on the cognitive function of older adults: a meta-analytic study. *Psychol Sci*, 14, 125–30.

Colcombe, S. J., Kramer, A. F., Erickson, K. I., Scalf, P., McAuley, E., Cohen, N. J., Webb, A., Jerome, G. J., Marquez, D. X. & Elavsky, S. 2004. Cardiovascular fitness, cortical plasticity, and aging. *Proceedings of the National Academy of Sciences of the United States of America*, 101, 3316–21.

Cracchiolo, J., Mori, T., Nazian, S., Tan, J., Potter, H. & Arendash, G. 2007. Enhanced cognitive activity – over and above social or physical activity – is required to protect Alzheimer's mice against cognitive impairment, reduce Aβ deposition, and increase synaptic immunostaining 2331. *Neurobiology of Learning & Memory*, 88, 277–94.

Debette, S. & Markus, H. S. 2010. The clinical importance of white matter hyperintensities on brain magnetic resonance imaging: systematic review and meta-analysis. *BMJ*, 341, c3666.

Erickson, K. I., Prakash, R. S., Voss, M. W., Chaddock, L., Hu, L., Morris, K. S., White, S. M., Wojcicki, T. R., McAuley, E. & Kramer, A. F. 2009. Aerobic fitness is associated with hippocampal volume in elderly humans. *Hippocampus*, 19, 1030–9.

Erickson, K. I., Raji, C. A., Lopez, O. L., Becker, J. T., Rosano, C., Newman, A. B., Gach, H. M., Thompson, P. M., Ho, A. J. & Kuller, L. H. 2010. Physical activity predicts gray matter volume in late adulthood: The Cardiovascular Health Study. *Neurology*, 75, 1415–22.

Erickson, K. I., Voss, M. W., Prakash, R. S., Basak, C., Szabo, A., Chaddock, L., Kim, J. S., Heo, S., Alves, H., White, S. M., Wojcicki, T. R., Mailey, E., Vieira, V. J., Martin, S. A., Pence, B. D., Woods, J. A., McAuley, E. & Kramer, A. F. 2011. Exercise training increases size of hippocampus and improves memory. *Proceedings of the National Academy of Sciences of the United States of America*, 108, 3017–22.

Erickson, K. I., Weinstein, A. M. & Lopez, O. L. 2012a. Physical activity, brain plasticity, and Alzheimer's disease. *Archives of Medical Research*, 43, 615–21.

Erickson, K. I., Weinstein, A. M., Sutton, B. P., Prakash, R. S., Voss, M. W., Chaddock, L., Szabo, A. N., Mailey, E. L., White, S. M., Wojcicki, T. R., McAuley, E. & Kramer, A. F. 2012b. Beyond vascularization: aerobic fitness is associated with N-acetylaspartate and working memory. *Brain and Behavior*, 2, 32–41.

Etnier, J. L., Nowell, P. M., Landers, D. M. & Sibley, B. A. 2006. A meta-regression to examine the relationship between aerobic fitness and cognitive performance. *Brain Research Reviews*, 52, 119–30.

Fabel, K., Fabel, K., Tam, B., Kaufer, D., Baiker, A., Simmons, N., Kuo, C. J. & Palmer, T. D. 2003. VEGF is necessary for exercise-induced adult hippocampal neurogenesis. *European Journal of Neuroscience*, 18, 2803–12.

Fiatarone Singh, M. A., Gates, N., Saigal, N., Wilson, G. C., Meiklejohn, J., Brodaty, H., Wen, W., Singh, N., Baune, B. T., Suo, C., Baker, M. K., Foroughi, N., Wang, Y., Sachdev, P. S. & Valenzuela, M. 2014. The Study of Mental and Resistance Training (SMART) Study-Resistance Training and/or Cognitive Training in Mild Cognitive Impairment: A Randomized, Double-Blind, Double-Sham Controlled Trial. *Journal of the American Medical Directors Association*, 15, 873–80.

Groves, J. O., Leslie, I., Huang, G. J., McHugh, S. B., Taylor, A., Mott, R., Munafo, M., Bannerman, D. M. & Flint, J. 2013. Ablating adult neurogenesis in the rat has no effect on spatial processing: evidence from a novel pharmacogenetic model. *PLoS Genetics*, 9, e1003718.

Holden, H. M., Hoebel, C., Loftis, K. & Gilbert, P. E. 2012. Spatial pattern separation in cognitively normal young and older adults. *Hippocampus*, 22, 1826–32.

Honea, R. A., Thomas, G. P., Harsha, A., Anderson, H. S., Donnelly, J. E., Brooks, W. M. & Burns, J. M. 2009. Cardiorespiratory Fitness and Preserved Medial Temporal Lobe Volume in Alzheimer Disease. *Alzheimer Disease & Associated Disorders*, 23, 188–97.

Kirk-Sanchez, N. J. & McGough, E. L. 2014. Physical exercise and cognitive performance in the elderly: current perspectives. *Clinical Interventions in Aging*, 9.

Landis, S. C., Amara, S. G., Asadullah, K., Austin, C. P., Blumenstein, R., Bradley, E. W., Crystal, R. G., Darnell, R. B., Ferrante, R. J., Fillit, H., Finkelstein, R., Fisher, M., Gendelman, H. E., Golub, R. M., Goudreau, J. L., Gross, R. A., Gubitz, A. K., Hesterlee, S. E., Howells, D. W., Huguenard, J., Kelner, K., Koroshetz, W., Krainc, D., Lazic, S. E., Levine, M. S., Macleod, M. R., McCall, J. M., Moxley, R. T., 3rd, Narasimhan, K., Noble, L. J., Perrin, S., Porter, J. D., Steward, O., Unger, E., Utz, U. & Silberberg, S. D. 2012. A call for transparent reporting to optimize the predictive value of preclinical research. *Nature*, 490, 187–91.

Lautenschlager, N. T., Cox, K. L., Flicker, L., Foster, J. K., Van Bockxmeer, F. M., Xiao, J., Greenop, K. R. & Almeida, O. P. 2008. Effect of physical activity on cognitive function in older adults at risk for Alzheimer disease: a randomized trial. *JAMA*, 300, 1027–37.

Lazarov, O., Robinson, J., Tang, Y., Hairston, I., Korade-Mirnics, Z., Lee, V., Hersh, L., Sapolsky, R., Mirnics, K. & Sisodia, S. 2005. Environmental Enrichment Reduces Aá Levels and Amyloid Deposition in Transgenic Mice. *Cell*, 120, 701–13.

Liu-Ambrose, T., Nagamatsu, L. S., Voss, M. W., Khan, K. M. & Handy, T. C. 2012. Resistance training and functional plasticity of the aging brain: a 12-month randomized controlled trial. *Neurobiology of Aging*, 33, 1690–8.

Lopez-Lopez, C., Leroith, D. & Torres-Aleman, I. 2004. Insulin-like growth factor I is required for vessel remodeling in the adult brain. *Proceedings of the National Academy of Sciences of the United States of America*, 101, 9833–8.

Macrae, P. G., Spirduso, W. W., Walters, T. J., Farrar, R. P. & Wilcox, R. E. 1987. Endurance training effects on striatal D2 dopamine receptor binding and striatal dopamine metabolites in presenescent older rats. *Psychopharmacology (Berl)*, 92, 236–40.

Meeusen, R., Smolders, I., Sarre, S., De Meirleir, K., Keizer, H., Serneels, M., Ebinger, G. & Michotte, Y. 1997. Endurance training effects on neurotransmitter release in rat striatum: an in vivo microdialysis study. *Acta Physiologica Scandinavica*, 159, 335–41.

Molnar, F. J., Hutton, B. & Fergusson, D. 2008. Does analysis using "last observation carried forward" introduce bias in dementia research? *CMAJ*, 179, 751–3.

Nature. 2014. *Nature Special: Challenges in irreproducible research* [Online]. http://www.nature.com/nature/focus/reproducibility/.

Nithianantharajah, J. & Hannan, A. 2006. Enriched environments, experience-dependent plasticity and disorders of the nervous system 2248. *Nature Reviews Neuroscience*, 7, 697–709.

Norton, S., Matthews, F. E., Barnes, D. E., Yaffe, K. & Brayne, C. 2014. Potential for primary prevention of Alzheimer's disease: an analysis of population-based data. *Lancet Neurology*, 13, 788–94.

Pantoni, L. 2010. Cerebral small vessel disease: from pathogenesis and clinical characteristics to therapeutic challenges. *Lancet Neurology*, 9, 689–701.

Pereira, A. C., Huddleston, D. E., Brickman, A. M., Sosunov, A. A., Hen, R., McKhann, G. M., Sloan, R., Gage, F. H., Brown, T. R. & Small, S. A. 2007. An in vivo correlate of exercise-induced neurogenesis in the adult dentate gyrus. *Proceedings of the National Academy of Sciences of the United States of America*, 104, 5638–43.

Podewils, L. J., Guallar, E., Kuller, L. H., Fried, L. P., Lopez, O. L., Carlson, M. & Lyketsos, C. G. 2005. Physical activity, APOE genotype, and dementia risk: findings from the Cardiovascular Health Cognition Study. *American Journal of Epidemiology*, 161, 639–51.

Prakash, R. S., Voss, M. W., Erickson, K. I. & Kramer, A. F. 2015. Physical activity and cognitive vitality. *Annual Review of Psychology*, 66, 769–97.

Prakash, R. S., Voss, M. W., Erickson, K. I., Lewis, J. M., Chaddock, L., Malkowski, E., Alves, H., Kim, J., Szabo, A., White, S. M., Wojcicki, T. R., Klamm, E. L., McAuley, E. & Kramer, A. F. 2011. Cardiorespiratory fitness and attentional control in the aging brain. *Frontiers in Human Neuroscience*, 4.

Prinz, F., Schlange, T. & Asadullah, K. 2011. Believe it or not: how much can we rely on published data on potential drug targets? *Nature Reviews Drug Discovery*, 10, 712.

Richard, E., Gouw, A. A., Scheltens, P. & Van Gool, W. A. 2010. Vascular care in patients with Alzheimer disease with cerebrovascular lesions slows progression of white matter lesions on MRI: the evaluation of vascular care in Alzheimer's disease (EVA) study. *Stroke*, 41, 554–6.

Robinson, A. M., Eggleston, R. L. & Bucci, D. J. 2012. Physical exercise and catecholamine reuptake inhibitors affect orienting behavior and social interaction in a rat model of attention-deficit/hyperactivity disorder. *Behavioral Neuroscience*, 126, 762–71.

Roig, M., Nordbrandt, S., Geertsen, S. S. & Nielsen, J. B. 2013. The effects of cardiovascular exercise on human memory: a review with meta-analysis. *Neuroscience & Biobehavioral Reviews*, 37, 1645–66.

Rovio, S., Spulber, G., Nieminen, L. J., Niskanen, E., Winblad, B., Tuomilehto, J., Nissinen, A., Soininen, H. & Kivipelto, M. 2010. The effect of midlife physical activity on structural brain changes in the elderly. *Neurobiology of Aging*, 31, 1927–36.

Ruscheweyh, R., Willemer, C., Krueger, K., Duning, T., Warnecke, T., Sommer, J., Voelker, K., Ho, H. V., Mooren, F., Knecht, S. & Floeel, A. 2011. Physical activity and memory functions: an interventional study. *Neurobiology of Aging*, 32, 1304–19.

Sahay, A., Scobie, K. N., Hill, A. S., O'Carroll, C. M., Kheirbek, M. A., Burghardt, N. S., Fenton, A. A., Dranovsky, A. & Hen, R. 2011. Increasing adult hippocampal neurogenesis is sufficient to improve pattern separation. *Nature*, 472, 466–70.

Salthouse, T. 2012. Consequences of age-related cognitive declines. *Annual Review of Psychology*, 63, 201–26.

Scarmeas, N., Luchsinger, J. A., Schupf, N., Brickman, A. M., Cosentino, S., Tang, M. X. & Stern, Y. 2009. Physical activity, diet, and risk of Alzheimer disease. *JAMA*, 302, 627–37.

Siette, J., Westbrook, R. F., Cotman, C., Sidhu, K., Zhu, W., Sachdev, P. & Valenzuela, M. J. 2013. Age-specific effects of voluntary exercise on memory and the older brain. *Biological Psychiatry*, 73, 435–42.

Smith, A. M., Spiegler, K. M., Sauce, B., Wass, C. D., Sturzoiu, T. & Matzel, L. D. 2013. Voluntary aerobic exercise increases the cognitive enhancing effects of working memory training. *Behavioural Brain Research*, 256, 626–35.

Smith, P. J., Blumenthal, J. A., Hoffman, B. M., Cooper, H., Strauman, T. A., Welsh-Bohmer, K., Browndyke, J. N. & Sherwood, A. 2010. Aerobic exercise and neurocognitive performance: a meta-analytic review of randomized controlled trials. *Psychosomatic Medicine*, 72, 239–52.

Sofi, F., Valecchi, D., Bacci, D., Abbate, R., Gensini, G. F., Casini, A. & Macchi, C. 2011. Physical activity and risk of cognitive decline: a meta-analysis of prospective studies. *Journal of Internal Medicine*, 269, 107–17.

Sparling, P. B., Howard, B. J., Dunstan, D. W. & Owen, N. 2015. Recommendations for physical activity in older adults. *BMJ*, 350, h100.

Stark, S. M., Yassa, M. A. & Stark, C. E. 2010. Individual differences in spatial pattern separation performance associated with healthy aging in humans. *Learning & Memory*, 17, 284–8.

Steiner, J. L., Murphy, E. A., McClellan, J. L., Carmichael, M. D. & Davis, J. M. 2011. Exercise training increases mitochondrial biogenesis in the brain. *Journal of Applied Physiology (1985)*, 111, 1066–71.

Strasser, B. & Pesta, D. 2013. Resistance training for diabetes prevention and therapy: experimental findings and molecular mechanisms. *BioMed Research International*, 2013, 805217.

Valenzuela, M., Bartres-Faz, D., Beg, F., Fornito, A., Merlo-Pich, E., Muller, U., Ongur, D., Toga, A. W. & Yucel, M. 2011. Neuroimaging as endpoints in clinical trials: are we there yet? Perspective from the first Provence workshop. *Molecular Psychiatry*, 16, 1064–6.

Valenzuela, M., Esler, M., Ritchie, K. & Brodaty, H. 2012. Antihypertensives for combating dementia? A perspective on candidate molecular mechanisms and population-based prevention. *Translational Psychiatry*, 2, e107.

Van Praag, H., Shubert, T., Zhao, C. & Gage, F. H. 2005. Exercise enhances learning and hippocampal neurogenesis in aged mice. *Journal of Neuroscience*, 25, 8680–5.

Voss, M. W., Heo, S., Prakash, R. S., Erickson, K. I., Alves, H., Chaddock, L., Szabo, A. N., Mailey, E. L., Wojcicki, T. R., White, S. M., Gothe, N., McAuley, E., Sutton, B. P. & Kramer, A. F. 2013a. The influence of aerobic fitness on cerebral white matter integrity and cognitive function in older adults: results of a one-year exercise intervention. *Human Brain Mapping*, 34, 2972–85.

Voss, M. W., Prakash, R. S., Erickson, K. I., Basak, C., Chaddock, L., Kim, J. S., Alves, H., Heo, S., Szabo, A. N., White, S. M., Wojcicki, T. R., Mailey, E. L., Gothe, N., Olson, E. A., McAuley, E. & Kramer, A. F. 2010. Plasticity of brain networks in a randomized intervention trial of exercise training in older adults. *Frontiers in Aging Neuroscience*, 2.

Voss, M. W., Vivar, C., Kramer, A. F. & Van Praag, H. 2013b. Bridging animal and human models of exercise-induced brain plasticity. *Trends in Cognitive Sciences*, 17, 525–44.

Waters, R. P., Pringle, R. B., Forster, G. L., Renner, K. J., Malisch, J. L., Garland, T., Jr. & Swallow, J. G. 2013. Selection for increased voluntary wheel-running affects behavior and brain monoamines in mice. *Brain Research*, 1508, 9–22.

Weinstein, A. M., Voss, M. W., Prakash, R. S., Chaddock, L., Szabo, A., White, S. M., Wojcicki, T. R., Mailey, E., McAuley, E., Kramer, A. F. & Erickson, K. I. 2012. The association between aerobic fitness and executive function is mediated by prefrontal cortex volume. *Brain Behavior and Immunity*, 26, 811–9.

Yaffe, K., Fiocco, A. J., Lindquist, K., Vittinghoff, E., Simonsick, E. M., Newman, A. B., Satterfield, S., Rosano, C., Rubin, S. M., Ayonayon, H. N., Harris, T. B. & Health, A. B. C. S. 2009. Predictors of maintaining cognitive function in older adults: the Health ABC study. *Neurology*, 72, 2029–35.

11

Depression and cardiovascular risk: exercise as a treatment

Bradley L. Stilger, Barry A. Franklin, Justin E. Trivax
and Thomas E. Vanhecke

A widely-cited review suggested that approximately 75% to 90% of the incidence of coronary artery disease is explained by conventional risk factors (e.g. hypertension, hypercholesterolemia, obesity, cigarette smoking, diabetes, obesity, sedentary lifestyle) (Kannel, et al., 2009). This has led to the delineation of other risk factors that may help to clarify the residual (10% to 25%) or unaccounted risk. Psychological factors such as anger, emotional distress, depression, and lack of social support have been implicated as precursors of acute cardiovascular events and may be potential targets for education, screening, and behavioral intervention (Tables 11.1 and 11.2) (Whooley and Simon, 2000; Kroenke, et al., 2001). Although the incidence of cardiovascular disease (CVD) due to psychological risk factors is small when compared with the above-referenced risk factors, it is significant given that psychological problems may exacerbate unhealthy behaviors that put patients at risk for concomitant endocrine, thrombotic, inflammatory, and autonomic stressors.

The World Health Organization's World Health Surveys showed that clinical depression results in a greater decrement in composite health scores than other chronic diseases such as angina, arthritis, or diabetes (Moussavi, et al., 2007). Depression has been found to precede myocardial infarction (MI) in up to 50% of all acute cardiac events (Ariyo, et al., 2000; Rowan, et al., 2005; Scherrer, et al., 2009), and patients with depression have a mortality risk at least three to five times greater during the first year following MI than patients without depression (Frasure-Smith, 1993; Frasure-Smith, 2000). Depression is also associated with an unfavorable cardiovascular risk profile in adolescents (Rottenberg, et al., 2014). The causal link between depression and increased cardiac mortality has not been fully elucidated; however, it has been reported that patients with depression are less likely to take prescribed cardioprotective medications or adhere to recommended behavioral and lifestyle interventions designed to mitigate cardiovascular risk (Schulz, et al., 2000; Ziegelstein, et al., 2000).

Physical Exercise Interventions for Mental Health, ed. Linda C. W. Lam and Michelle Riba. Published by Cambridge University Press. © Cambridge University Press 2016.

Table 11.1 *Patient Health Questionnaire: 2 Items**

Over the past 2 weeks, have you experienced any of the following feelings?
(1) Little interest or pleasure in doing things.
(2) Feeling down, depressed, or hopeless.

* If the answer is "yes" to either question, then refer for more comprehensive clinical evaluation by a professional qualified in the diagnosis and management of depression or screen with PHQ-9.

Table 11.2 *Patient Health Questionnaire-9 (PHQ-9)* Depression Screening Scales*

Over the past 2 weeks, how often have you been bothered by any of the following problems?
(1) Little interest or pleasure in doing things.
(2) Feeling down, depressed, or hopeless.
(3) Trouble falling asleep, staying asleep, or sleeping too much.
(4) Feeling tired or having little energy.
(5) Poor appetite or overeating.
(6) Feeling bad about yourself, feeling that you are a failure, or feeling that you have let yourself or your family down.
(7) Trouble concentrating on things such as reading the newspaper or watching television.
(8) Moving or speaking so slowly that others have noticed. Or the opposite – being so fidgety or restless that you have been more active than usual.
(9) Thought that you would be better off dead, or of hurting yourself in some way.

* Questions are scored: not at all = 0; several days = 1; more than half the days = 2; and nearly every day = 3. Add together the item scores to get a total score for depression severity. Screening scores that indicate a high probability of depression (≥ 10) should be referred for a more comprehensive clinical evaluation by a qualified treatment professional/plan. A positive response to question # 9 requires immediate follow-up with the patient and his/her referring physician.

This chapter examines the role of depression in the development of CVD in both apparently healthy and "at risk" populations, and its prognostic impact with specific reference to gene susceptibility, pathophysiologic factors, and varied treatments. Additionally, we review the potential benefits of structured exercise, increased lifestyle physical activity, and other complementary interventions (such as tai chi and yoga) in preventing and treating depression.

Risk, behavioral considerations, and pathophysiology

Cardiovascular disease and depression are associated with increased mortality, disability, and escalating healthcare costs worldwide. In 2012, 8 of the top 25 prescribed medications, ranked by total expenditure, were used in the treatment of CVD or depression (Agency for Healthcare Research and Quality, 2015). Depression is an independent risk factor for MI in individuals without known CVD, and a depressive disorder before or after MI confers a less favorable prognosis. One worldwide prospective study found that depression is one of nine modifiable risk factors that account for 90% of the risk of a first MI (Rosengren, et al., 2004). Another prospective cohort examination of 1000 patients found that participants with baseline depressive symptoms had a 50% greater rate of subsequent cardiovascular events than their nondepressed counterparts (Whooley, et al., 2008). Depression and other behavioral

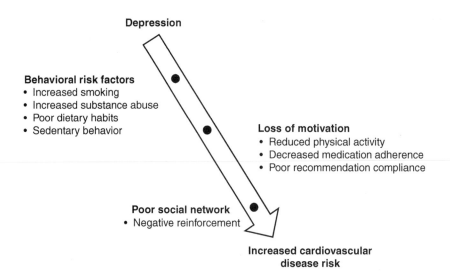

Figure 11.1 Pathway of depression leading to increased cardiovascular risk via behavioral changes.

risk factors tend to aggregate: depressed individuals are more likely to be habitually sedentary and overweight or obese, are more likely to smoke cigarettes, and are less likely to achieve abstinence from cigarette smoking (Figure 11.1) (Riba, et al., 2012). In contrast, effective treatment of depression may favorably influence some of these well-documented health modulators.

Some mechanisms by which depression may adversely impact the cardiovascular system include activation of inflammatory cytokines, elevated resting heart rates and blood pressures, endothelial dysfunction, and increased sympathetic nervous system activity (Figure 11.2) (Riba, et al., 2012; Nakatani, et al., 2005). Elevations in inflammatory mediators, proinflammatory cytokines and an upregulation of serum chemokines have also been reported in depressed individuals as compared with controls (Musselman, et al., 2000). Cytokines such as C-reactive protein, interleukin-6, and tumor necrosis factor have been shown to correlate with the severity of clinical depression as well as the development of CVD (Rethorst, et al., 2013; Duivis, et al., 2011). Another study found that depression was associated with higher levels of inflammatory biomarkers, though not necessarily the inverse (inflammatory biomarkers did not predict the development of depressive symptoms) (Duivis, et al., 2011). Finally, platelet reactivity is increased in individuals with depression, regardless of their cardiovascular history (Musselman, et al., 2000).

Effects of exercise and depression on cardiovascular physiology

Higher levels of cardiorespiratory fitness, typically expressed as $mLO_2/kg/min$ or metabolic equivalents (METs; 1 MET = 3.5 $mLO_2/kg/min$), and regular exercise

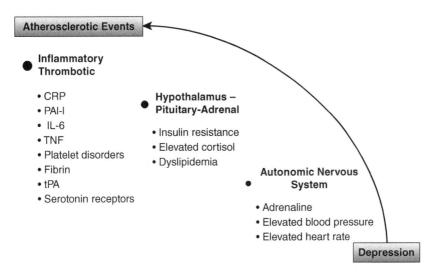

Figure 11.2 Proposed pathophysiologic mechanisms of depression as they relate to cardiovascular disease.

are associated with reduced all-cause and cardiovascular mortality. Individuals with higher levels of aerobic fitness often demonstrate lower resting heart rates, lower seated and supine blood pressures, and increased heart rate variability, measures that generally signify decreased cardiovascular risk. Beneficial changes in endothelial function, as indirectly measured by flow-mediated brachial artery vasodilation, are also observed in regular exercisers. These activity-related adaptations are considered cardioprotective and may serve to reduce the likelihood of coronary plaque rupture and/or lessen endothelial injury following an acute cardiac event.

In contrast, depression is associated with higher resting heart rates, elevated mean arterial pressures, reduced heart rate variability, increased systemic vascular resistance, and endothelial dysfunction (Figure 11.3) (Riba, et al., 2012; Musselman, et al., 2000; Pelletier, et al., 2009; Licht, et al., 2008). Depressed patients are also more likely to demonstrate lower cardiorespiratory or aerobic fitness during exercise testing. In patients with CVD, these variables may predict increased risk of nonfatal and fatal initial and recurrent cardiac events. Regular physical activity also has antagonistic effects, relative to depression, on cardiovascular reactivity. Accordingly, treatment of depression with structured exercise may serve to attenuate or reverse some of these physiological anomalies Riba, et al., 2012) (Table 11.3), decreasing the risk of CVD and its associated sequelae (e.g., heighted mortality).

Exercise as a treatment for depression in healthy individuals

Depression has the potential to cause adverse psychomotor changes, and many patients in the midst of a depressive period become more sedentary. Although few

Table 11.3 *Antagonistic Effects of Depression and Exercise on Traditional Cardiovascular Risk Factors*

Risk Factor	Effect of Depression	Effect of Exercise
Being overweight, obesity, metabolic syndrome	Promotes trends toward further weight gain and insulin resistance	Decreases weight via increased caloric expenditure, increases sensitivity to insulin
Current smoking status and likelihood of cessation	Makes individuals more likely to smoke, increases smoking frequency, and interferes with smoking cessation efforts	Individuals less likely to smoke, tend to smoke less frequently, and linked with improved smoking cessation rates
Lipids and inflammatory biomarkers	Worsens lipid profiles and increases inflammatory markers, some of which are atherogenic	Improves lipid profiles and reduces inflammatory markers
Hypertension	Elevates resting heart rate and blood pressure, and increases systemic vascular resistance	Lowers resting and exercise blood pressures, and lowers systemic vascular resistance
Physical activity	Depressed patients are usually more sedentary and less fit	
Medication adherence	Decreases rates of medication adherence	Increases medication adherence

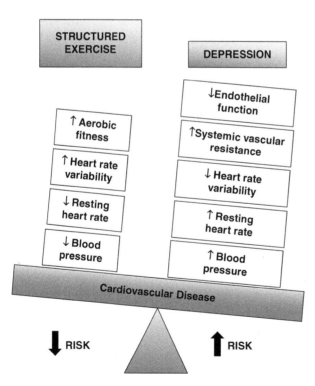

Figure 11.3 The oppositional effect of depression and structured exercise on cardiovascular risk.

data are available regarding the effect of structured exercise programs on depression in apparently healthy individuals, an early observational study that followed young adults through midlife found similar risk for the development of depression in both exercisers and nonexercisers (Cooper-Patrick, et al., 1997). In contrast, more recent prospective studies have shown structured exercise programs to be beneficial in inducing depression remission, preventing relapse, and improving depression severity scores. One study of 202 adults with depression compared the effectiveness of supervised exercise in a group setting, home-based exercise, or antidepressant medication (sertraline), versus placebo. At 16 weeks, remission rates were greatest in the medication and supervised exercise groups, 47% and 45%, respectively, followed by home-based exercise (40%) and placebo (31%) (Blumenthal, et al., 2007). Compared with placebo, individuals that continued the exercise regimen on their own demonstrated persistent benefits at 6-month follow-up. Another study stratified 80 depressed patients into one of four treatment groups of varying exercise intensity and frequency or to a control-placebo group (flexibility training); a 47% reduction in depression severity scores was demonstrated in the highest-level exercise group versus a 30% reduction at lower doses and 29% for controls, suggesting a dose-response relationship in using exercise as a treatment for depression (Dunn, et al., 2005). Similarly, a randomized, controlled trial in elderly subjects demonstrated the efficacy of exercise in alleviating depressive symptoms (Singh, et al., 2001), which was confirmed by a relevant meta-analysis demonstrating a moderate positive effect of regular exercise on depressive symptoms (Cooney, et al., 2014; Cooney, et al., 2013). Moderate exercise has also been shown to be an efficacious treatment for individuals with treatment-resistant major depressive disorder (Mota-Pereira, et al., 2011).

Risks of depression in patients with cardiovascular disease

Up to 65% of patients, many without pre-existing psychiatric disease, who have suffered a recent cardiac event, will develop symptoms of depression. Among this cohort, 20% will be diagnosed with a major depressive disorder (Lesperance, et al., 1996; Carney, et al., 1997), which is associated with a poorer prognosis than in patients without depression. Explanations for the increase in depression after cardiac events may include heightened sympathetic stimulation, dysregulation of serotonin receptors, immune system activation, or combinations thereof (Théroux, 2003). Post-event lifestyle changes including smoking cessation, adjunctive prescribed cardiac medications, dietary modifications, exercise-based cardiac rehabilitation, work-related uncertainties, and more frequent contact with physicians may also play a role.

Depressive symptoms often appear early after cardiac events such as acute MI, and the compounded impact invariably conveys a worse prognosis. One study showed that a major depressive disorder diagnosed at the time of hospital discharge for acute MI was associated with as great a six-month mortality risk as was the presence of left-ventricular systolic dysfunction (Frasure-Smith, et al., 1995). Up to a threefold increase in subsequent cardiac events, and heightened cardiovascular and all-cause mortality have been associated with post-MI depression (Melle and De Jong, 2004).

Depression is also very common in patients with congestive heart failure (CHF), and was documented in up to 36% of patients hospitalized with impaired myocardial contractility (Koenig, 1998). Patients with CHF and depression face a risk of death or hospital readmission rate up to double that of those without depression within the first year after the index hospitalization (Jiang, et al., 2001). One study of patients with depression and CHF demonstrated that those who remained depressed after a structured exercise regimen had nearly fourfold greater mortality than their counterparts who had improved with treatment (Milani, et al., 2011).

Relative to coronary revascularization, patients discharged after coronary bypass surgery with a major depressive disorder experience an increased risk of cardiac events as compared with nondepressed patients (Connerney, et al., 2001). It has also been demonstrated that depressed patients undergoing revascularization intervention for peripheral arterial disease experience a significantly increased risk of subsequent coronary events and/or contralateral vascular disease progression as compared with their nondepressed counterparts (Cherr, et al., 2008).

Despite the growing body of evidence demonstrating a modulating relation between acute cardiac events and depression, there is limited evidence to suggest that aggressive treatment of depression or related screening programs will favorably affect cardiovascular outcomes. Nevertheless, the American Heart Association recommends screening for depression in patients with coronary disease, as well as therapeutic treatment options such as structured physical activity, exercise-based cardiac rehabilitation, anti-depressant medications and/or cognitive-behavioral therapy (Lichtman, et al., 2008).

Adjunctive Exercise as Therapy for Depressed Cardiac Patients

Structured exercise, lifestyle physical activity, or both, may reduce symptoms in patients with CVD while simultaneously promoting decreases in LDL cholesterol and body mass index and increases in exercise capacity and HDL cholesterol. Several years ago, investigators reported that exercise-based cardiac rehabilitation decreased the prevalence of depression by 63% and that depressed patients completing cardiac rehabilitation also experienced a 73% reduction in mortality versus controls (Milani and Lavie, 2007). More recently, the UPBEAT (Understanding the Prognostic Benefits of Exercise and Antidepressant Therapy) study showed that both exercise and sertraline outperformed placebo in mitigating depressive symptoms while increasing heart rate variability (Blumenthal, et al., 2012).

The benefits of exercise have also been observed in elderly coronary patients, who are traditionally more difficult to enroll. When such patients are appropriately diagnosed and participate in exercise-based cardiac rehabilitation, improvements in depression, hostility, anxiety, and somatization have been observed (Milani and Lavie, 1998). A recent meta-analysis also concluded that cardiac rehabilitation programs in patients 64 years of age and older can significantly mitigate depressive symptoms after 16 weeks of treatment (Gellis and Kang-Yi, 1998).

Therapeutic exercise has also been shown to have antidepressive effects in stroke survivors. One study randomly assigned post-stroke patients into an exercise program that included strength, balance, and endurance training three times weekly for nine months. Patients in the exercise group demonstrated significant reductions in depressive symptoms as compared with those allocated to usual care (Lai, et al., 2006).

Exercise prescription for depression

Contemporary public health exercise guidelines recommend moderate-intensity physical activity for at least 30 minutes a day, 5 days per week (Garber, et al., 2011); vigorous activity for at least 20 minutes a day, at least 3 days per week, or combinations thereof (Haskell, et al., 2007). This exercise "dose" approximates an energy expenditure of 17.5 kcal/kg/week, which has been reported to be an effective treatment for mild-to-moderate depression; in contrast, more moderate energy expenditures (e.g., 7.0 kcal/kg/week) have been shown to be less effective or ineffective (Dunn, et al., 2005). This suggests that weekly gross energy expenditure is an important variable when considering exercise as a bona fide treatment for depression.

Healthcare professionals should aid the depressed patient in considering a variety of factors when beginning a structured exercise program (Pollock, 2001). An individual's previous behaviors (including avoidance tendencies), emotions (including fears about being judged), perceived participation/compliance limitations, support systems, interpersonal relationships, and co-morbid conditions should all be addressed. Patients may also express specific interests and/or preferences regarding exercise activities, and these should be incorporated, if possible, provided that they gradually meet the criteria for intensity, frequency, and duration. Maintaining an exercise program can be a challenge, and patients should be encouraged to rate and consider the activities that they would be most likely to adhere to and enjoy. Selected recommendations for assisting the patient in staying motivated and exercising regularly are briefly summarized in Table 11.4 (Riba, et al., 2012).

In addition to the minimum energy expenditure as suggested above, aerobic exercise programs should also be supplemented by resistance training at least two days per week (Haskell, et al., 2007). As compared with aerobic exercise, resistance training offers greater development of muscular strength, endurance, and muscle mass. It also helps in the maintenance of basal metabolic rate (to complement aerobic endurance training for weight management), promotes functional independence, and helps to prevent falls in the elderly (Garber, et al., 2011). Stretching exercises also may increase the ability of an individual to move joints through full range of motion, increase tendon flexibility, and augment muscular performance. Structured exercise programs should also be complemented by increased lifestyle physical activity such as walking during work breaks, gardening, using stairwells

Table 11.4 *Practical Recommendations for Maintaining Exercise Compliance*

- **Identify activities that you enjoy doing**. Identify physical activities that you enjoy and would be more likely to do, and consider when and how you'd be more likely to be consistent. Would you be more likely to enjoy a morning bicycle ride or a brisk walk after work?

- **Get your healthcare provider's and spouses' support**. Talk to your doctor, therapist, or other mental health professional, as well as your spouse. Ask for guidance and support if needed. Discuss with them how you envision an exercise program fitting into your treatment plan.

- **Set reasonable, obtainable goals**. Your initial goal does not have to be a plan to exercise vigorously five days per week. Think realistically about what you can and will do. Don't set unrealistic expectations.

- **Don't think of exercise as a chore**. Viewing exercise as just another "to-do" is a recipe for failure. Instead, try to view it as yet another intervention (such as therapy or medication) aimed at improving your overall health and fitness.

- **Address barriers to consistency**. Consider what's preventing you from exercising regularly. Problem solve: if money is an issue, consider something cost-free like walking. If you work better with a partner, recruit friends and family to join you in your program.

- **Be ready for setbacks**. Don't be too hard on yourself. Give yourself credit for even small steps in the right direction. If you miss a work-out day, get back on track the next day.

rather than elevators or escalators, and parking farther away from stores and walking (Franklin and Gordon, 2005).

Alternative therapies such as tai chi and yoga have also been suggested as treatments for depression. A pilot study involving a small number of subjects (n = 14) found that tai chi was effective in reducing depressive symptoms in older adults when compared with placebo (Chou, et al., 2004). A systematic review and meta-analysis concluded that tai chi may be associated with psychological benefits including reductions in stress, anxiety, and depression as well as increases in self-esteem, though the studies reviewed varied greatly in design and outcome measures (Wang, et al., 2010). Numerous other studies have shown that yoga is beneficial in treating depression (Pilkington, et al., 2005; Javnbakht, et al., 2009; Chen et al., 2010; Saeed, et al., 2010).

Beneficial effects of exercise on depression

The precise salutary links between exercise and depression remain unclear, but regular physical activity likely attenuates depressive symptoms in varied ways. Exercise releases neurotransmitters and/or endorphins that may lessen depressive symptoms, reduces antibodies and lymphokines that can worsen depression, and transiently increases body temperature, which can have a calming effect. Those who exercise regularly generally report increases in self-confidence, often a result of achieving even modest exercise goals. Such individuals may also report an improved sense of well-being and lower levels of stress and anxiety. Exercise also promotes socialization (thus reducing isolation), provides a distraction from negative ruminations, and may improve self-efficacy as well as physical appearance.

Conclusion

Depression is relatively common after an acute cardiac event, and the combination confers a poorer prognosis. Current data on the salutary effects of exercise on depression, cardiovascular risk factors, functional capacity and mortality identifies exercise as an effective multipurpose treatment option. Exercise-based cardiac rehabilitation, in conjunction with cardiovascular risk reduction, is an evidenced-based and efficacious treatment approach that may improve prognosis and psychological well-being.

Summary points

- Depression is a risk factor for initial and recurrent cardiovascular events.
- Depression is reported in up to 50% and 80% of patients prior to and following an MI, respectively.
- Depression is associated with increases in systemic inflammatory cytokines, sympathetic nervous system activity, resting heart rate and blood pressure, and platelet activation.
- Exercise induces antagonist and beneficial cardiovascular effects as compared with depression.

References

Agency for Healthcare Research and Quality 2015. 2012 Prescribed Drug Estimates: Top Prescribed Drugs by Total Expenditures. http://meps.ahrq.gov/mepsweb/data_stats/summ_tables/hc/drugs/2012/hcdrugest_totexp2012.shtml. Accessed March 17, 2015.

Ariyo, A. A., M. Haan, and C. M. Tangen. 2000. Depressive symptoms and risks of coronary heart disease and mortality in elderly Americans. *Circulation* 102: 1773–79.

Blumenthal, James A., Michael A. Babyak, P. Murali Doraiswamy, Lana Watkins, Benson M. Hoffman, Krista A. Barbour, Steve Herman, et al. 2007. Exercise and pharmacotherapy in the treatment of major depressive disorder. *Psychosomatic Medicine* 69: 587–96. doi:10.1097/PSY.0b013e318148c19a.

Blumenthal, James A., Andrew Sherwood, Michael A. Babyak, Lana L. Watkins, Patrick J. Smith, Benson M. Hoffman, C. Virginia, F. O'Hayer, et al. 2012. Exercise and pharmacological treatment of depressive symptoms in patients with coronary heart disease: results from the UPBEAT (understanding the prognostic benefits of exercise and antidepressant therapy) study. *Journal of the American College of Cardiology* 60: 1053–63. doi:10.1016/j.jacc.2012.04.040.

Carney, Robert M., Kenneth E. Freedland, Yvette I. Sheline, and Edward S. Weiss. 1997. Depression and coronary heart disease: a review for cardiologists. *Clinical Cardiology* 20: 196–200. doi:10.1002/clc.4960200304.

Chen, Kuei-Min, Ming-Hsien Chen, Mei-Hui Lin, Jue-Ting Fan, Huey-Shyan Lin, and Chun-Huw Li. 2010. Effects of Yoga on Sleep Quality and Depression in Elders in Assisted Living Facilities. *Journal of Nursing Research* 18: 53–61.

Cherr, Gregory S., Pamela M. Zimmerman, Jiping Wang, and Hasan H. Dosluoglu. 2008. Patients with depression are at increased risk for secondary cardiovascular events after lower extremity revascularization. *Journal of General Internal Medicine* 23: 629–34. doi:10.1007/s11606-008-0560-x.

Chou, K. L., P. W. H. Lee, and E. C. S. Yu. 2004. Effect of Tai Chi on depressive symptoms amongst Chinese older patients with depressive disorders: a randomized clinical trial. *International Journal of Geriatric Psychiatry* 19: 1105–7. doi:10.1002/gps.1178.

Connerney, I., P. A. Shapiro, J. S. McLaughlin, E. Bagiella, and R. P. Sloan. 2001. Relation between depression after coronary artery bypass surgery and 12-month outcome: a prospective study. *Lancet* 358: 1766–71. doi:10.1016/S0140-6736(01)06803-9.

Cooney, Gary M., Kerry Dwan, Carolyn A. Greig, Debbie A. Lawlor, Jane Rimer, Fiona R. Waugh, Marion McMurdo, and Gillian E. Mead. 2013. Exercise for depression. *Cochrane Database of Systematic Reviews* 9: CD004366. doi:10.1002/14651858.CD004366.pub6.

Cooney, Gary, Kerry Dwan, and Gillian Mead. 2014. Exercise for depression. *JAMA* 311. American Medical Association: 2432–3. doi:10.1001/jama.2014.4930.

Cooper-Patrick, L., D. E. Ford, L. A. Mead, P. P. Chang, and M. J. Klag. 1997. Exercise and depression in midlife: a prospective study. *American Journal of Public Health* 87. American Public Health Association: 670–3. doi:10.2105/AJPH.87.4.670.

Duivis, Hester E., Peter de Jonge, Brenda W. Penninx, Bee Ya Na, Beth E. Cohen, and Mary A. Whooley. 2011. Depressive symptoms, health behaviors, and subsequent inflammation in patients with coronary heart disease: prospective findings from the heart and soul study. *American Journal of Psychiatry* 168: 913–20. doi:10.1176/appi.ajp.2011.10081163.

Dunn, Andrea L., Madhukar H. Trivedi, James B. Kampert, Camillia G. Clark, and Heather O. Chambliss. 2005. Exercise treatment for depression: efficacy and dose response. *American Journal of Preventive Medicine* 28: 1–8. doi:10.1016/j.amepre.2004.09.003.

Franklin, Barry A., and Neil F. Gordon. 2005. *Contemporary Diagnosis and Management in Cardiovascular Exercise.* Handbooks in Health Care Company. Newtown, PA.

Frasure-Smith, Nancy. 1993. Depression Following Myocardial Infarction. *JAMA* 270: 1819. doi:10.1001/jama.1993.03510150053029.

Frasure-Smith, N., F. Lesperance, G. Gravel, A. Masson, M. Juneau, M. Talajic, and M. G. Bourassa. 2000. Social Support, Depression, and Mortality During the First Year After Myocardial Infarction. *Circulation* 101: 1919–24. doi:10.1161/01.CIR.101.16.1919.

Frasure-Smith, N., F. Lesperance, and M. Talajic. 1995. Depression and 18-Month Prognosis After Myocardial Infarction. *Circulation* 91: 999–1005. doi:10.1161/01.CIR.91.4.999.

Garber, Carol Ewing, Bryan Blissmer, Michael R. Deschenes, Barry A. Franklin, Michael J. Lamonte, I. Min Lee, David C. Nieman, and David P. Swain. 2011. Quantity and quality of exercise for developing and maintaining cardiorespiratory, musculoskeletal, and neuromotor fitness in apparently healthy adults: Guidance for prescribing exercise. *Medicine and Science in Sports and Exercise* 43: 1334–59. doi:10.1249/MSS.0b013e318213fefb.

Gellis, Zvi D., and Christina Kang-Yi. 2012. Meta-analysis of the effect of cardiac rehabilitation interventions on depression outcomes in adults 64 years of age and older. *American Journal of Cardiology* 110: 1219–24. doi:10.1016/j.amjcard.2012.06.021.

Haskell, William, I-Min Lee, Russell Pate, Kenneth Powell, Steven Blair, Barry Franklin, Caroline Macera, Gregory Heath, Paul Thompson, and Adrian Bauman. 2007. Physical Activity and Public Health: Updated Recommendation for Adults from the American College of Sports Medicine and the American Heart Association. *Circulation.*

Javnbakht, M., R. Hejazi Kenari, and M. Ghasemi. 2009. Effects of yoga on depression and anxiety of women. *Complementary Therapies in Clinical Practice* 15: 102–104. doi:10.1016/j.ctcp.2009.01.003.

Jiang, Wei, Jude Alexander, Eric Christopher, Maragatha Kuchibhatla, Laura H. Gaulden, Michael S. Cuffe, Michael A. Blazing, et al. 2001. Relationship of Depression to Increased Risk of Mortality and Rehospitalization in Patients With Congestive Heart Failure. *Archives of Internal Medicine* 161: 1849–56. American Medical Association: 1849. doi:10.1001/archinte.161.15.1849.

Kannel, William B., and Ramachandran S. Vasan. 2009. Adverse Consequences of the 50% Misconception. *American Journal of Cardiology* 103: 426–7. doi:10.1016/j.amjcard.2008.09.098.

Koenig, Horold G. 1998. Depression in hospitalized older patients with congestive heart failure. *General Hospital Psychiatry* 20: 29–43. doi:10.1016/S0163-8343(98)80001-7.

Kroenke, Kurt, Robert L. Spitzer, and Janet B. W. Williams. 2001. The PHQ-9. *Journal of General Internal Medicine* 16: 606–613. doi:10.1046/j.1525-1497.2001.016009606.x.

Lai, Sue-Min, Stephanie Studenski, Lorie Richards, Subashan Perera, Dean Reker, Sally Rigler, and Pamela W. Duncan. 2006. Therapeutic Exercise and Depressive Symptoms After Stroke. *Journal of the American Geriatrics Society* 54: 240–7. doi:10.1111/j.1532-5415.2006.00573.x.

Lesperance, Francois, Nancy Frasure-Smith, and Mario Talajic. 1996. Major Depression Before and After Myocardial Infarction: Its Nature and Consequences. *Psychosomatic Medicine* 58: 99–110.

Licht, Carmilla M. M., Eco J. C. de Geus, Frans G. Zitman, Witte J. G. Hoogendijk, Richard van Dyck, and Brenda W. J. H. Penninx. 2008. Association between major depressive disorder and heart rate variability in the Netherlands Study of Depression and Anxiety (NESDA). *Archives of General Psychiatry* 65. American Medical Association: 1358–67. doi:10.1001/archpsyc.65.12.1358.

Lichtman, Judith H., J. Thomas Bigger, James A. Blumenthal, Nancy Frasure-Smith, Peter G. Kaufmann, François Lespérance, Daniel B. Mark, David S. Sheps, C. Barr Taylor, and Erika Sivarajan Froelicher. 2008. Depression and coronary heart disease: recommendations for screening, referral, and treatment: a science advisory from the American Heart Association Prevention Committee of the Council on Cardiovascular Nursing, Council on Clinical Cardiology. *Circulation* 118: 1768–75. doi:10.1161/CIRCULATIONAHA.108.190769.

Melle, J. P. Van, and P. De Jonge. 2004. Prognostic association of depression following myocardial infarction with mortality and cardiovascular events: a meta-analysis. *Psychosomatic Medicine* 66: 814–22.

Milani, Richard V., and Carl J. Lavie. 2007. Impact of Cardiac Rehabilitation on Depression and Its Associated Mortality. *American Journal of Medicine* 120: 799–806. doi:10.1016/j.amjmed.2007.03.026.

Milani, R. V., and C. J. Lavie. 1998. Prevalence and effects of cardiac rehabilitation on depression in the elderly with coronary heart disease. *American Journal of Cardiology* 81: 1233-36.

Milani, Richard V., Carl J. Lavie, Mandeep R. Mehra, and Hector O. Ventura. 2011. Impact of exercise training and depression on survival in heart failure due to coronary heart disease. *American Journal of Cardiology* 107: 64–8. doi:10.1016/j.amjcard.2010.08.047.

Mota-Pereira, Jorge, Jorge Silverio, Serafim Carvalho, Jose Carlos Ribeiro, Daniela Fonte, and Joaquim Ramos. 2011. Moderate exercise improves depression parameters in treatment-resistant patients with major depressive disorder. *Journal of Psychiatric Research* 45: 1005–11. doi:10.1016/j.jpsychires.2011.02.005.

Moussavi, Saba, Somnath Chatterji, Emese Verdes, Ajay Tandon, Vikram Patel, and Bedirhan Ustun. 2007. Depression, chronic diseases, and decrements in health: results from the World Health Surveys. *Lancet* 370: 851–8. doi:10.1016/S0140-6736(07)61415-9.

Musselman, Dominique L., Ulla M. Marzec, Amita Manatunga, Suzanne Penna, Andrea Reemsnyder, Bettina T. Knight, Aimee Baron, Stephen R. Hanson, and Charles B. Nemeroff. 2000. Platelet Reactivity in Depressed Patients Treated with Paroxetine. *Archives of General Psychiatry* 57. American Medical Association: 875. doi:10.1001/archpsyc.57.9.875.

Nakatani, Daisaku, Hiroshi Sato, Yasuhiko Sakata, Issei Shiotani, Kunihiro Kinjo, Hiroya Mizuno, Masahiko Shimizu, et al. 2005. Influence of serotonin transporter gene polymorphism on depressive symptoms and new cardiac events after acute myocardial infarction. *American Heart Journal* 150: 652–8. doi:10.1016/j.ahj.2005.03.062.

Pelletier, Roxanne, Kim L. Lavoie, Jennifer Gordon, André Arsenault, Tavis S. Campbell, and Simon L. Bacon. 2009. The Role of Mood Disorders in Exercise-Induced Cardiovascular Reactivity. *Psychosomatic Medicine* 71: 301–7.

Pilkington, Karen, Graham Kirkwood, Hagen Rampes, and Janet Richardson. 2005. Yoga for depression: the research evidence. *Journal of affective disorders* 89: 13–24. doi:10.1016/j.jad.2005.08.013.

Pollock, Kenneth M. 2001. Exercise in treating depression: broadening the psychotherapist's role. *Journal of Clinical Psychology* 57: 1289–1300. doi:10.1002/jclp.1097.

Rethorst, C. D., M. S. Toups, T. L. Greer, P. A. Nakonezny, T. J. Carmody, B. D. Grannemann, R. M. Huebinger, R. C. Barber, and M. H. Trivedi. 2013. Pro-inflammatory cytokines as predictors of antidepressant effects of exercise in major depressive disorder. *Molecular psychiatry* 18. NIH Public Access: 1119–24. doi:10.1038/mp.2012.125.

Riba, Michelle, Lawson Wulsin, Melvyn Rubenfire, and Divy Ravindranath. 2012. *Psychiatry and Heart Disease: The Mind, Brain, and Heart.* Hoboken, NJ: John Wiley & Sons.

Rosengren, Annika, Steven Hawken, Stephanie Ôunpuu, Karen Sliwa, Mohammad Zubaid, Wael A. Almahmeed, Kathleen Ngu Blackett, Chitr Sitthi-Amorn, Hiroshi Sato, and Salim Yusuf. 2004. Association of psychosocial risk factors with risk of acute myocardial infarction in 11,119 cases and 13,648 controls from 52 countries (the INTERHEART study): case-control study. *The Lancet* 364: 953–62. doi:10.1016/S0140-6736(04)17019-0.

Rottenberg, Jonathan, Ilya Yaroslavsky, Robert M. Carney, Kenneth E. Freedland, Charles J. George, Ildikó Baji, Roberta Dochnal, et al. 2014. The Association Between Major Depressive Disorder in Childhood and Risk Factors for Cardiovascular Disease in Adolescence. *Psychosomatic Medicine* 76: 122–27. doi:10.1097/psy.0000000000000028.

Rowan, Paul J., Donald Haas, John A Campbell, David R. Maclean, and Karina W. Davidson. 2005. Depressive symptoms have an independent, gradient risk for coronary heart disease incidence in a random, population-based sample. *Annals of epidemiology* 15: 316–20. doi:10.1016/j.annepidem.2004.08.006.

Saeed, Sy Atezaz, Diana J. Antonacci, and Richard M. Bloch. 2010. Exercise, yoga, and meditation for depressive and anxiety disorders. *American Family Physician* 81: 981–6.

Scherrer, Jeffrey F., Katherine S. Virgo, Angelique Zeringue, Kathleen K. Bucholz, Theodore Jacob, Robert G. Johnson, William R. True, et al. 2009. Depression increases risk of incident myocardial infarction among Veterans Administration patients with rheumatoid arthritis. *General hospital psychiatry* 31: 353–9. doi:10.1016/j.genhosppsych.2009.04.001.

Schulz, Richard, Scott R. Beach, Diane G. Ives, Lynn M. Martire, Abraham A. Ariyo, and Willem J. Kop. 2000. Association Between Depression and Mortality in Older Adults. *Archives of Internal Medicine* 160. American Medical Association: 1761. doi:10.1001/archinte.160.12.1761.

Singh, N. A., K. M. Clements, and M. A. F. Singh. 2001. The Efficacy of Exercise as a Long-term Antidepressant in Elderly Subjects: A Randomized, Controlled Trial. *Journals of Gerontology Series A: Biological Sciences and Medical Sciences* 56: M497–M504. doi:10.1093/gerona/56.8.M497.

Théroux, Pierre. 2003. *Acute Coronary Syndromes: A Companion to Braunwald's Heart Disease*. Saunders. Philadelphia.

Wang, Chenchen, Raveendhara Bannuru, Judith Ramel, Bruce Kupelnick, Tammy Scott, and Christopher H Schmid. 2010. Tai Chi on psychological well-being: systematic review and meta-analysis. *BMC Complementary and Alternative Medicine* 10: 23. doi:10.1186/1472-6882-10-23.

Whooley, Mary A., Peter de Jonge, Eric Vittinghoff, Christian Otte, Rudolf Moos, Robert M. Carney, Sadia Ali, et al. 2008. Depressive symptoms, health behaviors, and risk of cardiovascular events in patients with coronary heart disease. *JAMA* 300. American Medical Association: 2379–88. doi:10.1001/jama.2008.711.

Whooley, M. A., and G. E. Simon. 2000. Managing depression in medical outpatients. *New England Journal of Medicine* 343: 1942–50.

Ziegelstein, Roy C., James A. Fauerbach, Sandra S. Stevens, Jeanine Romanelli, Daniel P. Richter, and David E. Bush. 2000. Patients with Depression Are Less Likely to Follow Recommendations to Reduce Cardiac Risk During Recovery from a Myocardial Infarction. *Archives of Internal Medicine* 160. American Medical Association: 1818. doi:10.1001/archinte.160.12.1818.